EXTREME R
WEIGHT LOSS
HYPNOSIS FOR WOMEN

2 BOOKS IN 1

HOW TO LOSE WEIGHT QUICKLY USING MEDITATION AND POSITIVE AFFIRMATIONS TO INCREASE SELF-ESTEEM AND HEAL YOUR BODY.

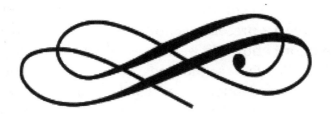

Eva Ruell

© Copyright 2020 - All rights reserved.

Table Of Contents

Introduction

Have you ever wished there was a means to give up smoking or eliminate weight forever and readily? Have you ever had difficulty sleeping and wanted that there was a direct answer? Have you ever wished you could unwind and have more significant memory retention while taking a check? Have you heard of having an ideal connection, being wealthy, and even with good wellness? While these are some pretty amazing objectives, this publication can help you take action in this way.

All of the information which you will need to unwind, restore your wellbeing, remove pain, or become capable of any of your needs is already inside you. This publication will show you how you can discover and use that magic strength, which lies dormant deep inside. All hypnosis is self-hypnosis. You devote nearly all your life to a hypnotizable state.

The definition of hypnosis is only open to tip. You're either free to advise or not. You accept matters, or you refuse them. If you're receptive to suggestions, you're in a more hypnotizable state. That's the foundation of communicating. The further you take and are amenable to tip, the more profound in hypnosis you're. You're being given hints always in almost every area you go and all that you do. This book is going to teach you how you can become mindful of many kinds of proposals you're being bombarded with daily. It occurs everywhere, in your grocery store, restaurants, on T.V. and any kind of media, on the job, while driving, in college, into the family, faith, nightclubs, the authorities, and practically everything else which you take part in.

As soon as you have become conscious of what's occurring, after that, you can take control of everything you reject or accept. You'll have the ability to use the knowledge of self-hypnosis to provide suggestions to advance in attaining your objectives. You are going to learn many strategies to hypnotize yourself permanently and quickly. A lot of these you are most likely doing at this time and are simply unaware of. You are going to learn the myths and roadblocks about alcoholism and also how to prevent them.

You'll have the ability to state your thought process to program yourself for success in each field of life, such as health, prosperity, relationships, joy, and a lot of other subjects. Simply take some opportunity to examine this book and follow the directions given. You may find that upon the conclusion of the book, you won't just have the capability to change just about any area of your life for the higher. Still, you are also going to be in a position to do precisely the same for the lives of your loved ones, friends, and nearest and dearest.

It's best to do this when you have a window of time ready for you to take care of this issue. You'll want at least thirty minutes of quiet time to handle these cravings, ideally an hour at most. You will be handling some pretty substantial matters, so making sure that you're relaxed and able to come back to reality before and after the hypnosis will make it all the better.

The effectiveness varies from person to person. It will help you, and, on average, a person loses about six pounds. You might lose more, but you might not lose as much as expected. If you're trying to lose a ton of weight, this might not help. But, if you're looking to help eliminate cravings in your life and live a healthier lifestyle, then this is definitely the right tool for you. It's a way to help you supplement your exercising plans, and with this, you'll be able to have an even better time when it comes to shedding those pounds fast. There are other benefits of using hypnosis for weight loss. The obvious big one is that you lose weight. That's the one people will notice. You'll start to shed those pounds, and you might lose more than you expected. It won't be significant, such as like fifty pounds or more, but if you want to help your body and allow yourself the benefits of being able to control the cravings to lose weight, then this is perfect for you.

Then there are the lasting benefits of it. These are the benefits that you'll get because of the hypnosis. When you're doing this, you'll be able to tackle those parts of your subconscious that think it's okay to eat when you're stressed, or it'll tell you to eat more than necessary. Sometimes, your mind can be your own worst enemy, and this is undoubtedly one of those times. With hypnosis for weight loss, you'll allow yourself to handle your body in a positive manner. If you do this, you'll actually enable yourself to control your cravings and desires through the use of hypnosis. It might seem crazy, but it is possible. It's a great way to take life by the horns, and by doing this, you'll be able to allow yourself the benefit of controlling the factors in your life, such as stress or how much you eat, and turning them around to give yourself a more positive image that will benefit you in ways you've never expected before.

How Does the Mind Work?

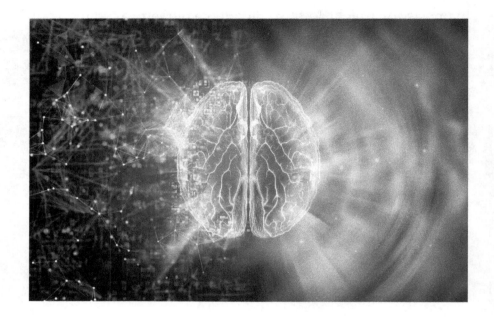

P erfect thoughts and ideal weight." The term may seem like a fantasy to you. Which is the ideal mind or ideal weight? They're the realistic conditions you'll be able to utilize as you pursue fat reduction. "Realistic?" You inquire. "How can anything be 'ideal,' let alone my burden and my ideas about my burden?" Well, recall what we said about the strength of believing and belief. Is it serving your curiosity to desire or hope for anything less than perfection on your own? Indulge us for some time as we clarify why you're able to think your mind and burden because "perfect."

Perfect fat is your weight that's ideal for you. It's the weight that's attainable and consistent with everything you need and precisely what you're ready to give yourself and accept yourself. More to the point, your ideal weight provides you with a healthy entire body, the human body which goes effortlessly, and also the one where you are feeling great about yourself and joyful. And what are ideal thoughts? You presently have a mind. It's flawless. But there can be a few ideas in that ideal thought of yours who are providing you with undesirable outcomes. There can be something that you keep in your mind, possibly habits or routines, which provide you with undesirable outcomes. However, you may use your ideal head to match your ideas to offer you precisely what you desire. It's possible to use your head to accomplish the bodyweight that you desire.

In the Twinkling of an Eye

Your current body is the consequence of your ideas and beliefs. You've behaved out these ideas and beliefs by your lifestyle, which generated your current weight. You haven't made any errors, regardless of what you may be thinking of yourself; instead, you've just experienced undesirable outcomes. These undesirable effects are an immediate effect of misaligned ideas and beliefs about yourself, which are very patterns of behavior or lifestyle. The Rapid Weight Loss Diet is all about utilizing your perfect thoughts

To align your ideas to provide you with the results you desire. You honestly can use your head to accomplish the bodyweight you desire. Let's examine a few of the learning which has occurred in your life, which has let you know where you're now together with your body weight. Do you wake up one afternoon, and you had been using the additional pounds? Or could it be a slow accumulation with time? Or perhaps you've understood nothing else as early youth. Whatever the situation, there are lots of factors that made your body:

- Food options

- Eating customs

- That the self-critic in you

- Economic history

- Psychological history

- Impact of household

- Impact of buddies

- Cultural heritage

These and several other variables were discovered in your life and eventually became the beliefs, which subsequently became routines of activity that generated your body. We'll be more specific. Notice that these aspects appear correct for you in your last years. In other words, consider what you did understand about your youth about eating and food.

What kinds of grocery stores did your household buy?

What foods did your kids cook, and were they typically ready?

Can you eat only at home or often grab food?

Have you been served fresh, healthy, high-calorie foods, or can you eat mainly processed and extremely processed foods, fried foods, and "junk" foods?

Was there an aware focus on nutrition, or has there been any irresponsible disregard for that which your household ate?

What did you find out about eating mindfully?

Were you educated that healthful food options led to healthy bodies?

Did anybody teach you how you can understand what's healthy food and what's not?

Are your meal selections based on which tasted or seemed high or priceless?

Can your loved ones or college instruct you about healthy lifestyles and audio nourishment, or has it been the "nutrition education" through TV advertisements and food makers' advertising?

What exactly did you learn as a kid? What're your beliefs about eating food, along with your entire body? Analyze your own socioeconomic or socio-cultural roots and see if they had an effect on the way and what you've learned to consume. Over thirty-five Years Back, sociological research pointed out weight issues in the working and lower class according to their intake patterns of what's been known as "poverty-level foods," like hot dogs, canned meats, and processed luncheon meats.

Cultural groups also have been analyzed to understand their nutritional patterns and meals, like eating with lard or ingesting a diet of fried and high-fat foods, which can lead to higher body fat loss. These influences can readily be accepted because they're "regular" into the category, of course. Then let's take a look at the teen years. During adolescence, are there some changes in your weight loss? Just as a boy, have you been invited to pile more food on your plate? "Look at him, consume! Certainly, he will develop to a large guy!" (There's a telling metaphor) Or are you currently admonished to eat? When you're a budding young woman, did a Smart girl take you under her wing and then with you that the marvel of menses and the wonderment of body modifications, such as the organic growth in body fat with all the evolution of breasts and broader hips?

Were you conscious during puberty, which unless the body improved body fat by 22 percent, it wouldn't correctly grow and create menses? Or was that "hushed up" within an awkward improvement? It was likely during adolescence which you heard there's a stigma involving obese individuals. Spend a couple of minutes writing down the aspects that appear to be accurate for you in your last years. Ponder the encounters and influences which are forming your body. In high school, the athletes at college sports have always been a healthful weight and are the cheerleaders and homecoming queens.

What ancient beliefs regarding your popularity and self-image could have formed from your social interactions in high school? What did you understand about physical activity, and what customs did you produce? Have you been introduced to physical activity as part of a healthy lifestyle, through family or sports outings of walks or hikes? Or was that the blaring TV a regular fixture, enticing everybody to the sofa? Next is a matter which most people have never been aware of throughout their development.

As you're growing up, has been that the attention of self-care based on trendy clothes, makeup, and hairstyles, or about healthful food, routine physical activity, along with spiritual and intellectual nourishment? What about today? Spend a couple more minutes writing down the aspects that appear to be accurate for you in the past couple of decades. What influences and experiences formed the ideas, which turned into the beliefs that turned into your body?

After high school, you moved away from the house. Suddenly you're no more captive to your family lifestyle. Can you be aware of your options, or can you start eating with blow off? If you input into a close connection, just what compromises or arrangements about foods and physical activity did you input into too? Most associations develop from similar pursuits, including food preferences and eating styles. In the end, the relationship comprises eating routines and tastes, which are a consequence of compromise.

Have your connections encouraged smart food choices and healthy eating? Maybe you've experienced pregnancy. Can you learn the way to get a wholesome pregnancy and then nourish a healthy infant within you? Or did you put in pounds? After giving birth, how did your lifestyle assist you in recovering your typical fat or suppressing it? If you were more active in the league or sports games, did your livelihood or family duties take priority and eliminate these physical fitness tasks from your regular? Can you correct exercise and diet so, or even did the fat begin to collect? Did an accident, injury, or disease happen that disrupted a standard physical action that has been supportive of healthy fat?

Because you can see, the way you got to where you're now was no crash. You heard from the folks about you--or you also consumed out of the surroundings --the best way to create food decisions, the way to eat, and the way to look after yourself emotionally and physically. Whether the thoughts you heard were tremendous and healthy or not so high and not as healthy, they became your own beliefs and eventually became you and the own human body because it is now. Bear in mind, and you didn't do something wrong; however, you need to experience the outcomes of eating and living, which have been consistent with your ideas and beliefs.

Through time, what's been your answer to individuals and their opinions about your weight loss, bad or good? Can you go out and purchase a fantastic pair of sneakers, or do you consume to facilitate psychological distress? Maybe you even heard the latter response in your youth.

Did your mom ever provide you with a plateful of food to comfort you when you're miserable? These are learned answers, and they may be unlearned and replaced with new answers and routines to make your ideal weight. Just ask, "Just how long does this happen?" We inform you, "In the twinkling of the eye," For the minute that you understand that you need it sufficient to get anything to possess it, it's completed. You've just altered the management of highly efficient energy in you and will redirect at figuring out how to attain the outcome which you need: your ideal weight.

Your Perfect Mind Relearning

It's simple to comprehend how you got or "heard" to contemplate over your ideal weight. And it'll be simple to create new decisions, to relearn new routines, and also to make new and much more healthful habits. How can we learn? We understand by mimicking another individual, analyzing books (such as that one) with different tools, and practicing the activities that create the outcomes we all seek. The best and lasting learning entails repetition and practice. The best way to practice is essential. Pretend for a minute that you're a violinist. You're searching for a grand symphony operation in New York.

Your piece includes five pubs, which are extremely difficult for your hands to perform appropriately. There are two ways that you practice. The first that is entirely ineffective would be to play with that steep fast, over and over and above, always playing precisely the very same mistakes, but trusting that your palms will play it properly. The next way to the clinic, which will always be active, would be to perform with the very, very slowly, mindfully "instruction" your hands the way to proceed, generating the "muscle " for the appropriate moves, before your palms have learned that the moves and may play with the whole segment correctly and in the appropriate pace with small if any, care focus. The critical point is that you're giving your focus on practicing correctly. By being aware of what you're practicing, and also the way you're practicing it, you're studying the new routines which are replacing the last routines.

Role of Human Mind in weight gain/loss

This chapter discusses in detail how a human brain can deceive you into gaining or losing weight. Triggers of overeating or underrating are discussed in this chapter. In order to attain optimal health, one should have a good relationship with food. Food should always be considered as a pleasant or joyful thing rather than giving it a name like food to reduce fat etc. This chapter will help you to overcome the negativity which you have for yourself so that you can live life to its fullest.

The brain does make you fat

Excess weight may feel like a thing of the belly, but your nervous system is among the major barriers to losing. What you feed, look and respond affects you whether or not you add weight. This is how the subconscious controls the body — and what you can do about it.

Anxiety fuels your needs.

Have a big presentation already come up, or are you about to have a challenging conversation with somebody you love? You should seek to control the discomfort; otherwise, you can catch yourself stopping the dinner otherwise preferred snack for a second. Sometimes referred to as stress feeding, fear causes this form of action and, when treated, may be counterproductive to the scale — both upward and downward.

Fear may have an overwhelming impact on the diet. Anxiety occurs differently in persons. Certain people will find themselves trying to regulate any ounce of food they consume, some may have the need to overeat, while some may lose their desire to eat completely.

Allowing negative to dominate

Within the head, the crystal-half-empty mentality may be challenging, but it often causes unhealthy habits of eating. Losing weight marketing is especially good for people who prey on the poor ways of thought that most people form about food.

The whole food industry is built to make consumers feel terrible for their health and make them believe they ought to waste all this money on a diet program that doesn't function.

Whenever the person's diet crashes, they feel bad for themselves and the process begins. People sometimes fault themselves for failing the diet, not the guy, when in fact it is. Before people get free of their eating habits, the body is hard to understand and everything that it offers, doesn't matter what big it might be.

Your brain turns dieting into fat preservation.

There are numerous misconceptions out there about weight reduction, but one aspect that is unequivocally real is that the brain avoids diet. Key brain cells actively prevent fat burning in the body when food is rare. A group of neurons in the brain coordinates appetite and energy spending and can turn on and off a switch to consuming or backup calories depending on what's in the environment available. We help us feed if food is abundant, and if food is unavailable, we transform our body into a survival mode to avoid from losing fat.

Depression triggers eating

Thinking processes causing obesity may be unconscious, but stress is an evident road to eating disorders. The weight gain is immutably related to the anxiety condition. Anxiety can significantly shift the culinary attitude and viewpoint. Depression feelings can manifest in excessive feeding or deprivation so what's important is resolving the head-on feelings. Recognizing what is going on is so crucial and finding professional treatment so that you really can take action not to allow stress to affect your well-being and weight.

Work destroys weight reduction targets

You can sense the cravings much more depressed than usual. And a brain under tension will indirectly weaken your attempts. If people feel uncomfortable regarding their bodies and eating patterns, the kinds of food they consume or the volume they consume can be unnecessarily limited. The body is created to live.

It doesn't realize why the human intentionally limits food, it only recognizes but it does not have sufficient, and it naturally slows down functions of the body, like metabolism, to save energy and to live. This physiological cycle often starts a primary urge to consume more to live, causing the individual to over-feed and struggle over food unconsciously.

Denying pleasure

Part of the weight-loss challenge is what products you choose to go there. If you're carelessly going for an apple because it's nice for you, however, it gives you a stomachache, why don't you make a move to eat a mango you'd like more?

Think about consuming an experience rather than a need. What that means is that by having the time to reflect on what you actually want to consume and make it a conscious activity, you allow yourself the chance to tune in and adapt to the nutritious meals that you would want to buy and enjoy, leaving you happy at mealtime.

Being judgmental

Will you feel a bad or a favorable connotation when you speak about a greasy burger and fries? How about a simple salad with hardly any treats? As we mature and start to assign various names to specific items, we start naming them accidentally — and sometimes, mindlessly —. Eliminating a 'good' behind such dishes and the 'evil' behind them will help shift the emphasis. "Food has little meaning, so feeding is not white and black. It has far less control over you, until the food has little moral obligation.

You don't even ask why

You remind yourself of something before you place the donut in your stomach. Is it food you desire — or anything else? "Enquire oneself if a meal is even whatever you need. People often crave comfort and support when eating without body hunger. It's fine to eat at a family party for selfish reasons, like cake, but you have to be capable to identify those signs and make a decision for yourself whether food is that you need or want or whether anything else will assist you accordingly.

Just to tap into gratitude

Humility can boost your well-being in several respects, but it's difficult to be thankful to oneself. Whenever an eating spree begins a cycle of shame, look at how incredible it is our brain and heart function to keep us healthy instead of throwing themselves a hard time. It gives sense why, if we build shortages by dieting, certain biological forces be in high gear to save our resources and lead us to search for high-calorie foods — or normally foods that we've resisted. What if we all quit dieting nonsense and chose to take control of our body and function through our appetite rather than battle it? Instead, in a range of body types and ages, we will find much healthier individuals who kept fairly healthy weights and enjoyed improved fitness.

Confidence won't support you

If you really can't turn your mind the correct way around? And do not be scared to ask somebody who is able to tackle something that delays your development, for assistance. Trying to break the dietary and food anxiety mental loop is challenging, it requires training and experience. A nutritionist who specializes in mindful eating as well as the – anti-diet method will assist you on the journey.

How to lose weight using your mind?

If you've ever attempted weight reduction, you realize that consuming nutritious food and exercising your body are essential elements of every weight-loss strategy. Yet have you learned that reaching or sustaining a balanced body structure exists both in the body and mind? In fact, if you've repeatedly tried to lose some weight but never succeeded or you lose the weight and then regain the weight (and then some!), your thoughts and beliefs — not your diet — are most likely holding you back. This is because the extra weight is a result of the state of mind or sentiment. And the main reason people struggle to lose weight is that they ignore to implement adjustments in their subconscious mind in order to support their conscious objectives.

How to Reshape Your Figure with Your Thoughts

Listen to your self-talk.

Self-respect and recognition of oneself are the key elements for reaching optimum weight. Yet, most individuals cannot lose weight when participating in body-shaming talk and actions.

It's crucial to learn if you spoke about yourself before attempting to lose weight. Whether you tell your body you dislike how it appears for much of your life or scratch your face in the mirror in frustration that someone used to do that to you, the subconscious mind would accept the emotional conditioning. You will reconfigure your subconscious mind by communicating with your body in a constructive, caring manner — the way you'd be communicating to an innocent kid.

Look in the mirror to see what the body likes. Touch the parts you want to change, and say, "Thank you for keeping me alive."

Make sure your body loses weight safely. Perform so every single day. Through time, the subconscious can comply with the urge to shed weight, actively.

Say affirmations.

Affirmations tend to reinforce your trust in the latest tale; you are designing the subconscious. When they are convincing, they do work well. Yet if you think, "I'm going to be 80 pounds thinner in a month," your amygdala won't accept it. Instead, try to say, "I become the super fit person that lives inside me! "And claim, 'I'm making good choices now that reflect my ideal weight.' You might also create a routine of voicing your comments. For example, you can smudge stagnant energy in your room or home, light candles, sit with your closed eyes, and say your statements three times in a row. Practice these two to three times a day. You may want to repeat another variation of your comments right before you feel sleepy when your subconscious mind is more open to advice. Remember, the affirmations have to be as if they had already manifested in the present tense. Affirmations will not trigger something to happen. They accept everything.

Try Tapping.

The Emotional Freedom Technique (EFT) or Tapping, helps match the subconscious mind with the expectations on an optimistic basis by resolving the unconscious feelings, habits, values, traumas, and more than that contribute to weight gain. You begin by stating your current restricting conviction preceded by expressing how you enjoy and support yourself while taping on different points of acupressure. For starters, you might claim, "I love and truly support myself even if I have a difficult time trying to lose weight." This removes stress levels in the body and can remove the negative emotions and values connected with the extra pounds, and you can break old patterns and recover.

Identify Your 'Trouble Thoughts'

Identify the thoughts that cause you trouble and fight to eliminate and alter it. Maybe if you look into a mirror, it's your inner voice. Or cravings when stressed out. Let them avoid knowingly by saying 'no' out loud. It may sound silly, but that simple action breaks your chain of thought and allows you to introduce something new or healthier. The best approach to do this is to count as many as you need from one to 100 times until the damaging thoughts fade.

Eat mindfully.

Research suggests that stress reduction — concentrated knowledge of your emotions, behaviors, and intentions — plays an important role in weight reduction in the long term when combined alongside certain weight loss approaches. Learn alertness when you cook and enjoy your food.

Seek to be aware of starvation and plenitude thoughts. Pay close attention to flavors, textures, and the munching as well as gulping actions of your food. Be conscious also of how the body sounds after consuming those foods.

This exercise will help lower binge and raise an understanding of behaviors that do not benefit the weight-loss goals. So, if you try to connect what you eat to how you feel, you're not going to have to eat normally to lose weight. It is going to happen mercilessly.

Also, your body composition and body image will be transformed when you learn from your mistakes about food as body-nourishment. When you link with your body and nurture it from an area of empathy and self-respect, the emotions focused on self-respect create in your body a metabolic environment conducive to ideal fat burning.

Address Yourself Like You Would a Friend

We are extremely tough on ourselves whenever it comes to beauty ideals and body image.

The expectations we set for ourselves are harsh. So, we should never have kept many of those requirements to our peers or loved ones. You receive the same consideration so kindness as everyone else; handle yourself like that.

Throw Out the Calendar

Patience is also important when you lose weight in a healthy and sustainable matter. Plus, if you focus on achieving genuinely actionable goals, such as taking 10,000 steps each day, and no need to get tangled up in a timeline of goals ahead.

Say "good-bye" to Energy Vampires.

One of the most striking things that have been observed in the relationships among both vampires and sensitive people is the discrepancy in their tendencies to gain weight. Your life and relationships represent your capacity to nurture yourself. If you are in a variant relationship where you constantly give and try to please some other individual, your efforts to lose weight will become in vain because you are using the energy of your vampire (which can be a state—not a person). This causes even more stress and cortisol and takes your own energy. As a result, you look out for sugar, carbs, and/or alcohol. And you will keep on gaining weight no matter what you do—even when you eliminate the carbohydrates because the weight acts as an extra layer of "self-protection.

Take a Breath

Taking a few minutes of stability at the beginning of your workout, or even at the beginning of your day, slowing down and simply focusing on the act of breathing can help you create your intentions, link with your body, and even lower the response to the stress of your body. Lie down with legs stretched and place one hand on your stomach and one on your chest. Inhale for four seconds, hold for two and then exhale through the mouth for six seconds. With each breath, the hand kept on your stomach should be the only one to rise or fall.

Designed to Eat

So why is it really so hard to reduce weight? The human body and brain are meant to eat explaining why weight loss proves so difficult for so many people. The factors of obesity are complicated. Obesity is not merely a laziness trait or an indicator of mental dysfunction. Therefore, hereditary and biological influences do not function in isolation but work with a variety of environmental variables on a permanent basis. Both the accessibility and persuasive advertising of unsafe food contribute to the epidemic of obesity.

CHAPTER 2:

The secret to lasting weight loss

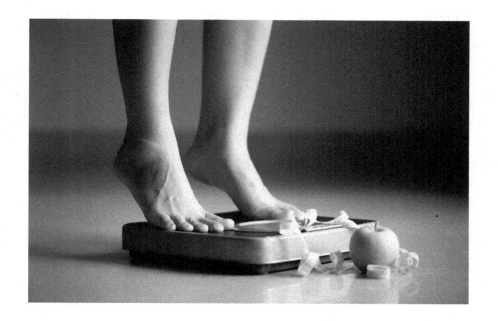

This script will help you maintain your weight loss. Weight maintenance is one of the hardest parts of weight loss, so many people can lose weight but struggle to keep the changes that they've made because of the challenges that naturally come when people have lost the weight and think, "Oh, the diet is over."

While you can make some dietary changes when you've lost weight and be less strict with yourself, you can never return to the bad habits that made you gain weight in the first place. Thus, hypnosis can give your unconscious brain the suggestions it needs to keep your weight steady once you have lost it.

Starter Script

You can stay healthy. Believe that you have the will to keep going. Sometimes, it gets hard, but you are resilient. You have created all the skills that you need to deal with the burdens that will try to drag you down. You are going to get through any hardship that comes your way because you believe in yourself, and you know how powerful your mind is. Your mind will guide you automatically when you are tired or are feeling defeated.

Now that you have taught it the skills it needs; it will try to further those skills even when you're at your most vulnerable. Repeat this message when you feel yourself slipping, "I am strong, and I can handle whatever life throws at me without returning to my old ways."

Give yourself breaks when you mess up. Do your best but be reasonable with yourself. Let yourself be human. You will not push yourself to do anything that will hurt you in the long run, even in the name of maintaining your weight. If you overeat, you will not turn to methods like purging or restriction.

You will continue to give your body what it needs, and you will not punish it. Instead of trying to make up for your slip-ups, you will choose to do better next time rather than torturing yourself over accidents because you'll always make mistakes no matter how long after you have lost the weight.

These messages will become part of you. You will listen to the notions that I have given because they will make you stronger. Let them settle into your brain and create new paths in your mind that will help you be successful at weight maintenance. Emerge from your trance and let yourself accept the suggestions that you have taken into your mind during this process.

Intermediate Script

Listen closely to the messages that I will give. These suggestions will encourage you to keep up the diligent work. Relax and let your thoughts calm. They will still make noise but focus on what you can do to improve your mind rather than silence it altogether. Let yourself be engaged in this process and find a new way of thinking.

When you have temptation, you will not give in. Think about all the things you can earn when you don't let temptation control you. Keep in mind the things you would lose if you gave up and let yourself go back to how you were. You don't want to go backward.

You want to continue forward using the momentum that you got from your weight loss. Let yourself improve and find victory beyond just weight loss. If you gain weight again, you'll have to start at square one, and that can be one of the least motivating places to be.

You've made it so far. There's no reason to go back. Don't be one of the people who fail to keep lost weight off. Choose to be one of the successful ones because failing will never make you feel good about yourself. If you can keep the weight off, you will prove to yourself that you are empowered to channel your mental energy into doing more extraordinary things.

If you gain the weight back, you will doubt your abilities and will stagnate yourself based on those doubts. Whatever weight you are doesn't matter, but it's the way you feel based on that weight that needs to change first and foremost. Funnily enough, having confidence that you lose and keep off weight is the thing you need to lose and keep off weight. You will keep it off if you remind yourself you will.

Remember all the people who are supporting you. Show them that you can succeed. Don't disappoint yourself and the people who helped you by self-sabotaging and returning to your old weight. You deserve permanent change for yourself more than others, but you still need to appreciate the help you got along the way.

Remind yourself of why you want to keep going and push yourself to maintain all the good habits you have created. Never quit bettering yourself. You have so much potential to unlock and embracing that potential and continuing to improve will help you resist reverting to your old self.

You're doing so well, so continue to do by embracing these suggestions. They will benefit you for years going forward and make it easier to maintain the good habits that you have created during your weight loss journey. Snap out of your trance and continue your day with the messages I have given to you.

Advanced Script

Use the suggestion in this script to reaffirm your goal to lose and keep the weight off. Take a big breath through your nose and close your eyes. Let yourself feel the inner stillness that allows you to focus on vital subconscious thoughts that you want to target. Breathe into a peaceful state, and let your mind emphasize these important messages that I will present to you right now.

You are so close to being where you've been working to be, so keep going. Continue bettering your brain in ways that have the most significant impact. When you boost your mind, you also nurture your body, so don't neglect your brain now that your body has changed.

You will get your beauty sleep. You will continue to get seven to eight hours of sleep per night because it is easier to keep up all the other good habits when you are well-rested. Your rest is not something that you will sacrifice. You will value it as a refreshing time for your body. Sleep is not an option. If you want to keep the weight off, you need it. Give yourself breaks, both mental and physical to keep in top shape.

Think of yourself in bed and imagine the calm you would feel as you sleep. Visualize your body, reinforcing itself for the next day. It is assembling an invisible armor around you that will protect you from your vulnerabilities and all the things that you can't foresee. Sleep builds that armor, and without it, you are prone to attacks. You'll feel more emotionally hungry if you don't sleep, so let yourself sleep even if you have a million things to do.

You will eat healthily. You cannot stop eating well just because you have lost weight. You will continue to make smart decisions about your diet. You will have foods that have nutrients and keep your body balanced. You will let yourself have treats, but you will not let those treats overrun your life and become coping mechanisms.

Visualize all the delicious meals that you will have. Imagine a table with heaps of colorful food. You can choose whatever foods you want. You can have a little bit of each food if you desire, but you can't eat it all without hurting yourself. If you eat it all, your stomach will grow, and you'll feel uncomfortably full and bloated. However, if you only choose what you need and a little of what you desire, you will feel great. You will have energy and peace of mind. You won't have to feel guilty when you do indulge.

You will continue to exercise. You'll let activities that make you happy continue to be a part of your life. You will enjoy the liberation you feel like your body moves and changes because of your workouts. Imagine your body moving smoothly and freely. Think of yourself as a feather gliding through the wind. You are not inhibited by anything weighing you down. You can push against the wind and steer where you are going.

Exercise gives you that lightness because it allows your body to do more incredible things. You will do greater things. You will push your body to do more things than you thought it could do. Your body is precious, so you won't force it to work out to the point of insanity, but you will let it have the rush of endorphins that come with being active.

You will keep the weight off. The excess weight will never be back on your body because you won't let it be. You will shove away all the things that threaten to bring the weight back. You will push through your fears and doubts to remain the weight you are happiest and healthiest at.

Think of how good you will feel when you have freedom from your weight. You'll feel calmer and more confident than ever when you have learned to love your body in all its sizes, but mainly its healthiest size.

Weight loss shouldn't be a fix-all. It won't cure your problems, but it can give you the state of mind you need to transform yourself from the inside out. Maintain your weight because weight loss is a tool you used to propel yourself forward in life. You will never be the size you hated again because you will do what it takes to maintain your weight loss.

You will let these suggestions into your subconscious. Permit them to take a permanent space in your head and serve as important reminders. They will solidify the progress you have made, and they will ensure that you lose weight for life. Your journey is not over. It never is, but you have made substantial progress, and you only must deal with the easy part of weight loss now— living your life and finding a new normal. Curate better habits and continue to force yourself to grow.

You will not let yourself stagnate. You will discover pursuits beyond weight loss. Weight loss will be just another part of your past, and weight maintenance will be a small but essential part of your daily life. You are more formidable and fitter than ever. Go out into the world and let yourself be happy, healthy, and feel less heavy. Emerge from your trance, and go live the good life!

Healthy Habits Are a Must

The habits you have make a difference in your weight loss, and these are many of the area's hypnosis will help you tackle, but you also need to be aware of the influence of these areas before you even begin hypnosis. The better handle you have on these parts of your life going into hypnosis, the more effectively your hypnosis will work. You need to have clear goals of what you expect of yourself. Determine how you want to handle each area better to promote the most success based on your personal experiences and needs.

Diet

Diet is probably the most essential addition to your hypnosis. All the research that has been done on hypnosis and weight loss has shown you need to have a good diet plan to do well with weight loss through hypnosis. The diet plan you choose is up to you, but there are many mistakes people make when trying to establish a diet. Often, they create unrealistic expectations for themselves, which inevitably leads to failure on their part. Be honest with yourself when you are planning your diet. Know what you'll be able to stick to, and know what parameters would drive you too crazy to handle in the long-term.

Keep a balanced diet. You need to have balance no matter what diet you choose, which means you need to maintain a variety of foods in your diet plan. Sure, eating a calorie-restricted diet plan of only candy will, in theory, lead to weight loss, but that diet plan would not be conducive to long-term change. You would become deficient in a variety of vitamins and minerals, and your body would practically beg you to eat other foods.

You'd end up eventually breaking your diet and returning to your old habits. The pounds would all go back on, and all that time you spent eating just one candy would be wasted. If you have the nutrients that you need, you are less likely to have those intense cravings that derail you from progress and make you feel like a failure.

Don't over restrict your food. When you become limiting with your diet, that's when it becomes hard to stick to it. There's no need to cut out your favorite foods. If you love potato chips, you don't need to cut them out altogether. Try to eat less of them, but you don't need to say, "I will never eat a potato chip again," because that is unrealistic. You aren't going to be able to resist them for the rest of your life.

Make changes that allow flexibility and that you can continue long past when you've lost all the weight you want to lose. It would help if you were trying to make lifestyle changes, not temporary ones. Successful diets don't have an end date. They continue for the rest of your life. That may sound grim, but once you change your habits, it won't feel so awful, especially if you make livable changes.

Carbs are not evil. For whatever reason, diet culture has furthered the idea carbs are bad for you. Yes, simple cards like sweets and white bread are not as nutritionally dense as other foods, but whole grains should be a vital part of your diet, and you should allow yourself to have simple carbs occasionally too.

Your body needs carbs to function because carbs are what fuel your brain. When you don't eat carbs, you may feel worse, and you will probably crave them because your body instinctually knows what it needs. Thus, instead of trying to cut carbs out, try to eat more complex carbohydrates like brown rice, wheat bread, or whole wheat pasta.

Fat isn't evil either. Since the 1980s, the diet industry has demonized fat, maybe even worse than carbs. Again, this rhetoric is inaccurate. While trans fats and saturated fats should be limited, your body does need fat. Fat is what your body uses to energize you between meals when you have burned through your carbs.

Fat also pads your organs and protects them. When you don't have enough fat, your body will begin eating muscles, including your heart! Low-fat diets can harm your body. Aim to include polyunsaturated fats and monounsaturated fats into your diet.

Proteins are also vital. These keep your muscles healthy, and they also have a myriad of diverse functions around your body. Aim to eat lean proteins like chicken or lean fish. Alternatively, you can eat plant-based proteins like soybeans (or tofu) or combine starch and legume/ seed to make a full protein (i.e. rice and beans). You'll want to eat proteins several times throughout the day because protein cannot be stored in your body, which is why trends like intermittent fasting can leave you feeling worse than if you were to have smaller meals throughout the day.

Don't forget your micronutrients! Vitamins and minerals are essential to your health because they keep your bodily functions such as vision and digestive health going. They also make sure you can use your muscles and that your heart can beat properly. They are part of all your systems, and you can be sure to get them through fruits and vegetables. Try to eat produce that is of a variety of colors and types to ensure that you get all the vitamins and minerals you need for your body to work as it should.

When you have a healthy diet, you will feel better all-around in your life. Plus, you will be taking the steps that you need to further your weight loss. Strive for satiety rather than trying to cut several foods out of your diet. You don't need to eat only vegetables and protein to be healthy. You can eat everything, but you merely have to change the way you eat those things. Incorporate more "good" things rather than eliminating all the "bad." Stop villainizing food. There aren't good or bad foods. You can have them all. Some foods are more nutritious than others while you should eat others in moderation.

Exercise

Exercise is another excellent way to promote a healthy lifestyle that you need for weight loss. Physical activity is a great mood booster that can help you feel better in your skin. It also allows you to replace fat with muscle so that you can tone your body.

When you exercise, you combine the powers of your mind with the capabilities of your body, and you build yourself up. Exercise is not just about your body, which is something that people don't always realize. Some physical activity allows you to be in a better headspace and to feel all-around better about yourself and your condition. The health benefits of exercise are extensive. By just adding a little bit of exercise a day, you can better your cardiovascular health. Even just an additional fifteen-minute walk can make you less likely to have heart disease. Further, it reduces your blood pressure, which makes you more resistant to stress. Some studies indicate that active people can reduce their risk of conditions like diabetes and cancer. Plus, being regularly active increases your immune function, making you less prone to illness in general. When you are more active, you'll probably feel better even if you can't see the changes in your body right away. People who exercise often get better quality sleep and can sleep longer, which is incredibly important to your health. You also feel mentally better when you exercise and are less depressed and anxious because of the feel-good endorphins that exercise sends through your body. Best of all, people who exercise live longer. You can't go wrong with exercise!

You don't need to start crazy workouts to be healthy. Find ways to enjoy exercise. You don't have to be a star athlete to reap the benefits of exercise. Anyone can improve their lives by just adding a little more activity. It doesn't have to be an organized workout either. Dancing in your living room or going for a bike ride through a park also counts even though they don't feel as scary as more intense activities. Do what makes you feel good and you'll be able to stick to it. You can build up to more workouts later if you are so inclined. When you live a more active life, you become happier and healthier. You also can lose weight when you add in more activity. Exercise can improve your life experiences in so many ways you won't realize until you add it consistently to your life.

Sleep

Sleep is one of the most critical parts of your overall health. People who get more sleep have better health outcomes, both physical and mental. The impacts of sleep on your health carry many of the same benefits of exercise. People who get more sleep tend to live longer. They also have better heart health. When you sleep, you feel less stressed and can deal with anxiety better. You feel ready to take on the world rather than wanting to ignore all your issues.

You are less moody when you sleep, so it is easier to keep your spirits up and avoid the pull of emotional eating. If you make no other change in this eBook, change your sleep because when you aren't sleeping, your body struggles to function. Driving when you are sleep deprived can be as bad as driving drunk, which shows how dangerous not getting sleep is!

Additionally, you tend to reach for foods that take less energy to prepare, which usually means junk food that does not fill you because it is nutritionally empty. Alternatively, leptin is the hormone that makes you feel full. When your body sends leptin through your body, you know you've had enough food; however, when you are tired, your body doesn't produce as much leptin.

Thus, with the rush of ghrelin and little leptin, you are hungrier and don't feel as satiated regardless of the amount of food that you are eating. Further, when you are tired, you are more emotional, so you might eat food to deal with feelings because you are too exhausted to cope with them in any other way. You'll want the nutritionally empty foods you habitually choose. As a result, getting sleep is a crucial part of managing your body's hunger cues and cravings.

Do not underestimate the value of sleep. Sleep is something that people often try to skip. They think that they are too busy to take eight hours from their schedule for sleep. If you want hypnosis to work and to lose weight, you need to take care of your body and get your rest in. If you don't, you will not be in the headspace to respond well to treatment.

Your body will fight against you even more than it would normally. You have time to sleep. Watch less TV, and you'll probably quickly find a little more time to sleep. We're all busy, but when we get to sleep, we can be more productive during the hours that we do work. Tired people take forever to get anything done.

Mental Health

To make lasting changes, you need to address your mental health. Hypnosis can help you improve your mental health, but it targets specific areas, so if you have issues beyond your weight that you need to address, find ways to manage them. Don't let your emotional wounds keep hurting you. It is time to move on and get better.

Share your past hurts with a friend, loved one, or a therapist. Don't run away from your problems. It would be best if you faced the things that hurt you and owned up to the things that fuel your inability to lose weight. Be kinder to yourself. Stop beating yourself

CHAPTER 3:

How to use meditation to beat food cravings

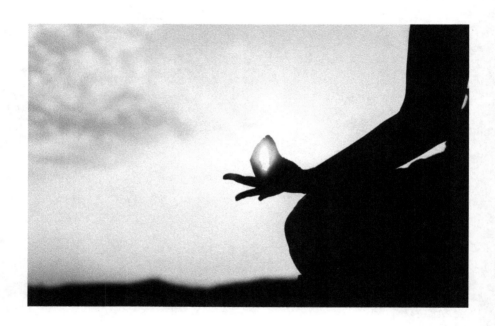

When it comes to rapid weight loss, meditation is one of the techniques that act like secret weapons. Studies conducted on meditation and mindfulness have shown that these exercises are linked to weight loss. They not only boost an individual's awareness but also banish belly fat and lower stress levels. Having an attentive mind can help you avoid binge or emotional eating.

What is Meditation?

Meditation must not be a difficult technique. If you are a beginner, take only five minutes when you wake up to clear your mind before you start off your day. You just need to close your eyes and focus your mind on your goals as you breathe in and out. As you breathe, don't let your mind wander, and if this happens simply guide it back without making any judgment.

What is the Connection between Meditation and Weight Loss?

Meditation is known to be an effective tool for weight loss. It aligns the unconscious mind with the conscious mind in order to facilitate changes that we want to make in our behaviors. Such changes may include avoiding unhealthy foods by altering them with healthier foods. It is important that your unconscious mind becomes engaged in the change process because it is where the weight-gaining, poor habits such as emotional eating are cultivated. Through meditation, you will be able to become more aware of your surroundings and will be able to overcome your unhealthy habits.

But there is even a more immediate effect of mediation. It can reduce the level of stress hormones in the body. Hormones like cortisol give the body signal to store more calories. If you have high levels of cortisol moving through your system, it is going to be difficult to cut down weight even if you are eating healthy foods. Most of us are stressed in most cases, but it takes only 25 minutes of meditation three times in arrow to reduce the effects of stress.

In 2016, a study that was conducted by Texas Tech University found that increased relaxation, attention, body-mind awareness, calmness, and brain activity result from just a few sessions of meditation. The study also suggested that your self-control could increase with daily meditation. The researchers found that the brain is most affected by meditation, which means that with a few minutes of meditation, you will be able to pass by that ice cream when feeling stressed.

How to Start Meditating for Weight Loss

Even without training, anyone who has a body and mind can practice meditation. For most of us, the most challenging aspect of meditation is getting time. You can start with as little as 8 to 10 minutes a day.

Ensure that you are able to access a quiet place for meditation. If you have children or other people around you, you may need to squeeze time when they are not awake or after they have left the house to avoid distractions. You may even practice your mediation while in the shower.

Once you are in a place of silence, take a comfortable position. You can either lie down or sit in a position that makes you feel at ease.

Start meditating by putting your focus on your breath. Watch the way your stomach or chest rises and falls. Feel the air that you breathe in and out of your mouth. Listen keenly to the sounds around you. This should be done for 2 or 3 minutes until you begin feeling relaxed.

Next, do the following steps:

- Take in a deep breath, and hold for a few seconds

- Slowly breathe out, and repeat the process

- Breathe in a natural manner

- Observe the way your breath enters your nostrils, influence the movement of your chest, and moves your stomach.

- Continue focusing on the way you breathe in and out for about 8 to 10 minutes

- Your mind may begin to wonder, which a normal occurrence is. Just acknowledge this and return your attention back to the process

- As you wrap up, reflect on your thoughts, and acknowledge how you can easily bring your mind together

Benefits of Meditation on Weight Loss

Below are the incredible ways that meditation can help you achieve daily weight loss:

Meditation reduces stress

With meditation, you will feel calmer as well as have a stress-reducing impact on your body. With endless roles in life including work, children, and home activities, it is not surprising that you may be overwhelmed, which may contribute to increased stress. Unfortunately, these stressors affect your body by producing more cortisol, a stress hormone that affects the levels of sugar and insulin in the body. As a result, the hormone causes weight gain. Studies have revealed that meditation activates a relaxation response, regulating the nervous system and, in turn, lowering the cortisol levels.

With a few minutes of deep breathing and conscious relaxation, you will be able to obtain the cortisol-lowering benefits as well as your overall stress levels.

Meditation promotes a focus on intention

Often, meditation techniques involve focusing on specific goals or concepts. Meditating on cutting down weight streams your energy, thoughts, and intentions to a particular goal. In this case, you submit to the intentions by revealing your goals to the world, which makes both your conscious and subconscious mind to be aware of the goal that you want to lose some weight. The outspoken intention will stay with you for a long while, enabling you to achieve your weight loss goal both consciously and subconsciously, and dodging all possible distractions.

With meditation, you will learn conscious eating

With daily meditation, you will be able to boost your levels of mindfulness and awareness. This can allow you to live in the moment and always focus on what you are doing in the present. The process of meditation can help you gain an increased sense of awareness of actions and thoughts, thus helping you to think twice before you have taken action. Rather than enabling your cravings to take over you, you will develop the power of controlling your mind, thus handling your cravings with greater intention and awareness. When you are ready to eat, your awareness will make it easier to recognize the textures and flavors of the food you are eating, instead of taking them for granted.

Meditation stabilizes mood hormones

Common daily stressors and activities can affect the way your system operates normally and may throw your hormones out of normal functioning. Apart from keeping your cortisol and adrenaline levels regulated, meditation goes further than this. The technique for relaxation releases both oxytocin and serotonin hormones, which boost your moods and ensure your hormones remain stable.

Meditation regulates sleep

Lack of sleep may hinder your weight loss progress. You see, by having a deep sleep, your cortisol levels will rise, which in turn will sabotage your progress in losing weight. Also, when you lack sleep, ghrelin, a hunger signal hormone, is also produced in plenty, thereby increasing your chances of eating more for weight gain. With meditation, you will be able to balance the circadian rhythms that promote quality sleep. Meditation increases the levels of melatonin, a hormone that also determines and controls when you sleep.

How to Make Sure that Meditation Works for You

If you want to include meditation in your rapid weight loss hypnosis, it is important that you make it simple. Meditation should help you recover from any stressful event, not become a source of it. That is why you need to consider the three easy ways highlighted below, which you can incorporate in your daily mediation.

Consider a Mantra That Can Help You Lose Weight

A mantra refers to a phrase that one repeats to focus their mind on mediation and bring them to a relaxation state. A mantra can give help you identify something to focus on as you meditate. Although it is very helpful to many people, a mantra is not a must in meditation. You don't need to force yourself to use one if you don't find it helpful or if it does not make you feel natural. However, in case you choose to use one, you need to repeat it as you inhale as well as when you exhale. Some of the common mantras used include "I am at peace with myself," "I am loved," or "I can do this."

Follow Your Breath to Avoid Stress

As you meditate, try to count your inhales 4 times and exhales 8 times. Remember that meditation is a process that is aimed at reducing stress; if these counts do not feel natural, you should deviate from them. Every time you meditate, always try to increase the number of exhaling and inhaling counts. Do not feel stressed if it takes longer to reach 8 counts. Just keep in mind that lengthening the exhale will greatly affect your health as you will be able to calm down.

Consider a Guided Meditation

If you are not able to practice meditation alone, you should consider a guided process. This includes websites, phone apps, podcasts, and recordings that can help you connect with experts who guide you on how to meditate.

How to Create a Meditation Space at Home

You may find it easier to practice meditation on a daily basis to motivate your weight loss process. Creating and incorporating meditation accessories and organizing the right space might help you throughout the practice. Some of the equipment to get started including:

Essential Oil Diffuser

Aromatherapy is considered an effective calming tool for the body, which is very helpful during meditation. An essential oil diffuser can help you create a relaxing environment in order to reap the benefits of the essential oils. Additionally, the diffuser always shuts off when the water runs out; thus, you can meditate as long as you like.

Bluetooth Earbud Headphones

Don't have enough space to practice your meditation? You may consider wireless headphones, which you can to wherever you go.

The headphones can sync up with Android and iPhones devices, which you can use to listen to your best-guided mediation without bothering those close to you.

A Meditation Filled Cotton Pillow Cushion

A meditation cushion can give you the comfort to find a point of relaxation. The cushion will relieve you from stress, especially after having a prolonged sitting period. It has the perfect density and height to sit through for hours of meditation practice.

Meditation That Will Burn Your Fats

Our bodies were designed to burn fat. It is the way that they provide the body with energy when we haven't given it enough through the foods we eat. We require more energy when we workout, so our bodies will burn more fat during these processes.

Though it can sound so simple on paper, it will be rather challenging to always include these things in our lives.

This meditation is going to help guide you through the journey of getting the body you want, with a visualization exercise to help you see your goals laid out clearly. Listen to this first when you are in a relaxed position in case you become calm to the point of sleep.

After you know how you react, you might include this when you are doing yoga or another form of light exercise to help keep you grounded and relaxed.

Meditation and Daily Habits

People become emotionally attached to food from infancy through adulthood. Children sometimes get rewarded with snacks or treats for healthy behavior; adults can be treated to dinner. There are so many celebrations across the year from Christmas, Halloween, Thanksgiving, birthdays, and Valentine's Day. All these celebrations are food-focused, and as people eat together, they feel good and happy.

It has also been proven that an aroma of a special kind of baked cake can create an emotional connection memory that will last throughout someone's lifetime. Some foods are for nourishment, but others we take just for comfort, depending on how they make us feel. Whenever the brain reacts and feels pleasure for a particular food within our reach, most of the time, we will grab it and eat it. During this time, the brain releases a chemical called dopamine, the process feels perfect, and if we equate the feeling with food, then the outcome will be negative.

High body mass index (BMI) can be linked to emotional problems like anxiety, depression, and stress. Those emotional issues can make one overindulge after a rough day at the office as a reward for a good feeling. Some people use junk food as a coping mechanism when they hear bad news. This habit can be only be improved by the use of meditation exercises to deal with one's emotions, stress, or anxiety. As the practices continue and you pay close attention to your breath and allocate more time for thinking.

Tackling Barriers to Weight Loss

There are so many barriers to weight loss from personal, to medical, to support system and emotional health. Meditation, if incorporated, will bring fruitful and healthy results. Dedication to overcome the challenges and to be focused on achieving your goals is significant. There are so many distractions, especially before you start tour weight loss routine.

It takes discipline and resilience to manage a healthy loss program. We need to give weight loss the priority it deserves. Also, we need to realize the existence of the said barriers and their contribution toward our goal. The barriers will determine our successes and failures.

<u>Set realistic goals</u>

When you set goals, ensure that they are attainable, specific, and realistic. It is effortless to work on realistic goals and achieve them for better results. If the goals are unrealistic; however, the success rate will be low since one will be discouraged. For instance, when starting with meditation, you can start with as little as five minutes a day and gradually increase it daily until you reach the maximum time like sixty minutes.

The same applies to lose weight during the meditation process. You can start focusing on losing a few pounds each week and gradually increase until you reach your goal. As you set goals, however, realize that it is not your fault if they do not work out as you had planned, do your best and keep your focus.

Always be Accountable

Once you have decided to commit to meditation for weight loss, don't shy away from sharing your plan with your support system and family. It is to ensure that the people you share with also reinforce the commitment and form part of the support system. That way, they will feel part of the program and give support whenever there is a need. You can also use apps for reminders and timings; this way, you have a backup plan whenever you forget.

You can also use motivational bands whenever you achieve a milestone set. Being accountable makes you enjoy your successes, acknowledge your failure, and appreciate your support system.

People thrive when they feel responsible for something, especially for something beneficial to their well-being.

Modify Your Mindset

Your thinking needs to be modified in the sense that you be keen on the information you are telling yourself. Ensure that your mind is not filled with unproductive and negative thoughts, which will bring you down or discourage you. Do not be scared of challenging your thoughts and appreciate your body image.

Your mindset determines your thinking and in turn, creates a sense of appreciation or rejection. Our weight loss largely depends on our mindset; do you believe you can do it? If you think you have all it takes, then absolutely nothing will prevent or stop you.

Manage Stress Regularly

Having a stress management technique should be part of one's daily routine. You need to develop a healthy stress-relieving mechanism that can help you live a stress-free life. Understand that meditation is a stress reliever in its own right as it helps calm the mind and soothes the body.

It can be used to manage stress and its benefits fully utilized to live a more productive life. Be able to handle stress efficiently. Stress is not healthy for the mind.

If not handle, it can cause emotional problems and makes one irrational, moody, or violent. Be your own boss when managing your stress.

Be Educated About Weight Loss

As you embark on meditation for weight loss, be educated about how it works; that way, weight loss will not be a struggle.

You will be able to handle failed attempts as well as appreciate the progress made.

You will be able to know what you have been doing wrong and decide on the best meditation exercise for you.

If you have misleading information, then your general progress may be inhibited

Weight loss need not be too expensive; neither does it require a costly gym membership or enrolment in a costly meditation class. There are various self-practice meditation exercises that you can comfortably do at home. There are various meal plans and diets that may work for others though they may not offer long-term solutions or lasting behavior changes. Have the right information that you need. Don't be misled by anyone posing that they are professionals in that field. Also, do not hesitate to do research online and compare notes. From there, you will be able to come back with something that works for you.

CHAPTER 4:

What is Hypnosis?

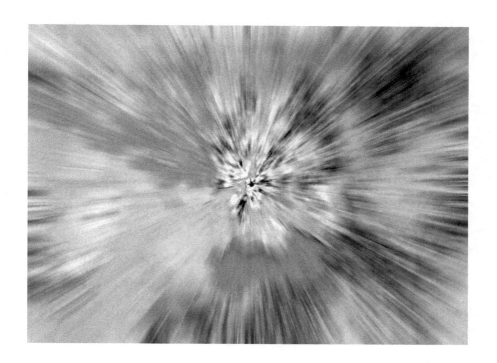

Hypnosis is a state of understanding of focus and concentration. There are two theories about how hypnosis works. The "country" theory implies that subjects enter a different condition of consciousness. The "on-state" concept says that hypnosis isn't an altered state of consciousness. Instead, the topic is responding to a proposal and actively engaging in the semester; instead of under the control of the hypnotist there are hypnosis methods. Among the very common is that the procedure, which entails keeping a constant stare until the eyes shut at a bright object. You're more when you've entered the state of hypnosis suggestible and more inclined to be more amenable to creating changes. Entering into a trance, relaxed state of consciousness Once a trance, the hypnotist will provide verbal ideas, for example, "if you awaken, you will feel more inspired" or even "you won't drink alcohol." Some argue that hypnosis might help recover repressed memories, treat dependence, cure allergies, and decrease depression and anxiety. Hypnosis is focus and responsiveness to tips. You are inclined to be amenable to creating positive behavioral changes.

We actually enter hypnosis each day without even thinking about it. Hypnosis is not like the things we see in Hollywood. You will not be a mindless drone. Nor will you mindlessly follow absurd commands. Instead, you will be able to use hypnosis to improve learning and to embed new lessons into your subconscious mind. Have you ever said to yourself, "I am going to lose weight"? Yet, a few weeks later you realized that you made that decision but still weighed the same, or even more? This is because you made a decision with the conscious mind, the part that is temporal and acts in the moment, rather than the subconscious mind.

In hypnosis, we are precisely the opposite of what Hollywood portrays. Like in meditation, we are more focused, goal-directed, and intuitively aware. Like an old-time cassette tape, you can record over the messages and the negative behavioral patterns of the past. This is why we will not be giving up anything in this first session. As you add new designs and new lessons to your life, you will naturally and intuitively replace old patterns.

There are several new habits that you will add to your life in this first session. First, you will add food to your diet. You will add nutrient-rich foods that are the source of natural energy and health. If you do this each day for a week, you will find that you will effortlessly eat less of the unhealthy things that may have been a part of your life. You will also add a new method of eating. The result will be recording over old patterns that, in the past, have been destructive. You will also add new activities to life and increase your daily physical activity.

The first step is to learn how to enter a state of hypnosis. For beginners, the easiest way to do this is to use guided relaxation.

In fact, because guided relaxation is a great way to manage stress, it will be your first new skill for managing weight. Many of our unhealthy patterns come from emotional reactions to stress. Most people never take the time, like you are doing today, to learn how to practice this skill.

So, by going through this necessary process you will have already added a tool that can be useful to you. Relaxation is a way of entering hypnosis because in a relaxed state we are open to new lessons and are comfortable considering new options. There is no right or wrong way to experience this. Begin by getting comfortable in your chair. In a few minutes, you will be very relaxed. However, you will always be attentive, able to hear my voice, and aware of your surroundings. You might listen to outside noises, but these will not distress you. In fact, they will reassure you that you are exactly where you need to be, doing exactly what you need to be doing.

Now that you have found a comfortable place to still the body and the mind, begin by scanning your body. Anywhere you are carrying the tension of the day in your muscles, simply let those muscles relax. Pay attention to the small muscles of the brow and around the eyes. Let them relax as well. Often, tension is held in tissues of the jaw. You can even allow these muscles to relax. As you relax, notice that you're breathing becomes slower and more natural. As you listen to the quiet in the room or hear the distant sounds of others outside of the room, give yourself permission to enjoy this time of developing a sense of deep relaxation.

As your hands rest on your lap, let them feel very relaxed, very heavy, and very calm. Again, scan your body and relinquish any remaining tension. Relax any residual tension held in the shoulders, back, or legs. Now, notice that your breathing is slower and calm. In just a few moments, your heart rate has even slowed. This necessary process of physical relaxation can also be used to still the mind. Do not worry if your account has been wandering or thinking. After all, this is what brains do. Imagine yourself under a clear blue sky. You can imagine that you are in a place you have been to before, would like to go, or a situation entirely of your own creation. In the sky, there is a single white puffy cloud, gently drifting towards the horizon. As it floats, send all of your thoughts, cares, and concerns into that cloud. Watch the cloud move farther and farther towards the horizon, until it disappears altogether. Now, both your body and mind are completely relaxed. If any other thoughts surface, just allow them to drift towards the horizon after that puffy cloud.

What is Self-Hypnosis?

The only significant difference between hypnosis and self-hypnosis is that in the first one, the operator and the subject are two different people, while in self-hypnosis the operator and the subject coincide in the same person.

This shared experience can be of great value to both, as it will unite them mentally and emotionally and promote love and mutual respect.

It is also a fact that learning is more comfortable and faster when done with another person.

Ask your partner to hypnotize you using a procedure similar to the one we used in the second session. Then practice the self-hypnosis exercise for a few days. Ask your partner once again to hypnotize you and reinforce hypnotic suggestion. Practice it again.

The number of times it is necessary to reinforce the procedure depends entirely on you. If you practice the daily self-hypnosis exercise, one or two reinforcement sessions will be sufficient.

But what about those who have no one with whom to share the learning experience of self-hypnosis? What can they do? How can they learn?

The Sense Spiral

This technique was developed by Betty Erickson, the wife of the famous psychiatrist and hypnotherapist Milton Erickson. It consists of stimulating all sensory perceptions to provoke a saturation (and therefore a relaxation) of the conscious.

First, focus your attention on a specific point at eye level or slightly above it. With your eyes open or closed, start by stating (aloud or in thought) 5 sentences that describe your visual experience ("I see); then five sentences describing your hearing experience ("I hear), then five sentences describing your kinesthetic experience ("I feel...").

Then repeat the same sequence, but with 4 sentences, then 3, then 2, then only one per direction.

Steps to Enable Self-Hypnosis

You would need to feel physically confident and secure to start the cycle. Seek to use a quick calming method.

Choose an item on which you can concentrate your eyes and mind – hopefully, this item would include you gazing upward directly on the wall or ceiling in front of you.

Free your mind of all thoughts and only concentrate on your goal. Obviously, this is hard to do, so take your time and let your emotions leave you.

Become mindful of your pupils, talk of making your eyelids heavy, and shutting gradually. Concentrate on breathing while your eyes shut, breathe in a deep and even manner.

Tell yourself every time you breathe out, you'll relax more. Slow your breathing, and let each breath relax deeper and deeper.

Use your mind's eye to visualize a gentle movement of an object up and down or sideways. Maybe a metronome's hand or a pendulum-something that has a normal, long, yet steady movement. See the object sway back and forth in your mind's eye or up and down.

Softly, gradually and monotonously start the countdown from ten in your mind, saying after each count, 10 I'm relaxing. '9 I'm calming etc.

Believe, and remember that you will have reached your hypnotic state when you finish counting down.

It is the time when you enter the hypnotic condition to reflect on the specific messages you've written. Focus on each statement-see it in the eye of your mind, repeat it in your thoughts. Relax and keep focused.

Relax and clear your mind before getting out of your hypnotic state once again.

Count steadily but energetically to 10. Reverse the process you used when you were counting down to your hypnotic state before. Use some positive messages, as you count, between every number. '1, I'll feel like I've had a full night' sleep when I wake up'... etc.

When you hit 10 you feel fully awakened and reborn! Let your conscious mind slowly catch up with the day's events and continue to feel refreshed.

Leave your worries aside.

It is possible to use self-hypnosis to solve virtually any type of problem and also to broaden your consciousness and connect with your innate superior intelligence and creative ability. By using self-hypnosis for the latter purpose, hypnosis can be transformed into meditation.

Self-hypnosis can also be used in those moments when you feel the need for a higher power to intervene in some situations; then, it becomes a prayer. The subtle differences between these forms of self-hypnosis lie in the way thoughts are guided once the state of consciousness itself has been altered, that is when the alpha state has been reached.

What a fantastic tool is self-hypnosis! It transports us to another state while we are comfortably and quietly sitting with our eyes closed, thinking about a specific objective. But using self-hypnosis in this sense is not easy to achieve since it requires a prolonged period of preconditioning in a hypnotic or auto hypnotic state. Such preconditioning is similar to that used for diet control, but the indications are different; it will be necessary to devise the techniques and suggestions for this case.

And it also requires practice, a lot of practice. Do not forget my words, time and effort will be rewarded with the results. Develop your discipline and stick to it; the results will be a real success.

Hypnosis for Weight Loss

In terms of weight loss, you already know the standard professionals: doctors, dietitians, personal trainers, and even psychological state coaches. But maybe you haven't thought of a hypnotist yet. Facts have proven that the utilization of hypnosis is different, and people take risks in weight loss. Greg Gorniak, a clinical and medical hypnotist, practicing in Ontario, said that sometimes, all other final efforts are tried and failed before it can pass.

But it's not that others control their thinking and let themselves do some exciting things in a comatose state. Kimberly Friedmutter, a hypnotherapist and author of Subscious Power, said: "Mind control, which is against your will, is the biggest misunderstanding of hypnosis." Due to how the show business portrays hypnotists, people are pleased to ascertain that I'm not wearing a black robe or swinging my watch from a sequence."

Can Hypnosis Help Lose Weight?

According to Malian Colman, the chairman of the Australian Association of Hypnotherapists (AHA), hypnosis can bring good results to customers trying to find weight loss assistance. However, she acknowledged that the virtual circle belt isn't for everybody. "(Virtual circle belt) works well in some people, but weight loss is complicated, and people's motivations for eating or overeating could also be very different. The therapist will work with the client to spot the matter for excellent hypnosis."

Lyndall Briggs, president of the Australian Association of Clinical Hypnotherapists (ASCH), said that she has been using hypnosis to scale back her clients' load over the years and has succeeded in hypnosis treatment. Still, she believes that a size suitable for all treatments isn't a fair idea. She said: "Different methods serve different customers."

Professor Clare Collins, a spokesperson for the Australian Association of Nutritionists (DAA), said that surprisingly. There are few studies on hypnosis and weight loss, which she attributed to "the disconnect between science and practice." She noted that past research results are mixed and difficult to realize because you can't blindly test subjects.

She added that a comprehensive review published in 2014 by Liverpool John Moores University reviewed previous research and results. The study's entire finding is by combining hypnotic drugs with traditional weight management strategies and using them continuously (rather than one time), some people enjoy hypnosis. However, the review found that anesthesia isn't valid for everybody, and hypnosis is considered to favor only those who are willing to accept advice.

Collins said that hypnosis could affect negative self-talk and shortcut self-destruction in the diet for those that respond well;

it can help overweight people become symptoms of past trauma. Collins emphasized that before all folks rushed so far, hypnosis alone was never enough. "There could also be other cognitive-behavioral therapies that are more suitable for a few individuals than other individuals (hypnosis), know what a healthy diet is, change eating habits, and exercise. You cannot just place your hopes on hypnosis."

Surprisingly, many scientific studies specialize in the effect of hypnosis on weight loss, many of which are positive. Original research completed in 1986 found that overweight women using hypnosis procedures lost 17 pounds, while women who had to concentrate on the diet lost 0.5 pounds. In the 1990s, a meta-analysis of hypnotic weight loss found that subjects who used hypnosis lost twice the maximum amount of weight as those that didn't. A 2014 study found that ladies using hypnotic drugs can improve body weight, BMI, eating behavior, and even improve body image.

But this is often not good news: A 2012 Stanford University study found that a few quarters of individuals couldn't hypnotize in the least. Contrary to popular belief, it had nothing to do with their personality. On the contrary, some people's brains don't seem to figure that way. "If you're tough to daydream, often hooked into books or watching movies, and do not think you're creative, then you'll be one among the people with poor hypnosis," Dr. Stan said. Georgia said that this not only helped her lose excess weight but also helped her maintain her weight. Six years later, she was happily maintaining weight loss, and infrequently checked again with a hypnotist therapist.

Who Should Try Hypnosis to Lose Weight?

The perfect candidates are those that enforce a healthy diet and exercise plan because they can't obviate bad habits. He said that stepping into bad habits (such as eating an entire bag of potato chips rather than stopping once you are full) may be a sign of a mental problem.

Friedman says that your subconscious mind is where your emotions, habits, and addiction are. Moreover, since hypnosis is aimed toward conscious people and unconscious people, it's going to be simpler.

Research analysis from 1970 found that hypnosis's success rate reached 93%, requiring less treatment than psychological and behavioral therapy. "This leads researchers to believe that hypnosis is the best method for changing habits, ways of thinking, and behavior," Friedmutter said. Hypnosis therapy doesn't need to be used alone.

What Do I Expect In Treatment?

The meeting time and method may vary, counting on the doctor. For instance, Dr. Cruz said that her treatment usually lasts 45 to 60 minutes, while Friedman believes that weight loss patients need 3 to 4 hours. But generally, you'll lie down, close your eyes and relax, and let the hypnotherapist guide you through specific skills and suggestions which will assist you in achieving your goals.

Friedman said: "The idea is to coach people to maneuver in a healthy direction but from an unhealthy direction." I used to be ready to identify mental obstacles that caused the customer to interrupt faraway from their [health] original blueprint through the customer's history. Even as we learn to abuse our bodies with food, we will learn to respect them. "No, you'll not giggle sort of a chicken, nor will you confess any profound secrets." Gorniak said: "You can't fall under a hypnotic state or be told or do something against your will." "If it violates your values or beliefs, you'll not take actions that supported the knowledge provided during the trance."

Gorniak added that, on the contrary, you'll feel deeply relaxed while still knowing what you're talking about. He said: "People in a hypnotic state will describe it as between awake and deeply asleep." "They are fully controlled and may stop the method at any time because you'll hypnotize once you prefer to do so. Teamwork to realize personal goals." In fact, the number of coaching sessions required depends entirely on your response to hypnosis. Dr. Cruz said that some people might only see one to three results, while others may have eight to fifteen meetings. Again, it's not going to work for everybody.

How Does Hypnosis Feel?

Forget everything you see in movies and on stage; therapeutic hypnosis is closer to healing than circus tricks. Dr. Stan said: "Hypnotherapy is a collaborative experience, and patients should understand things and feel comfortable at every step." For those that are worried about being deceived into doing strange or harmful things, she added, even under hypnosis, if you do not want to do something, you will not roll in the hay either. She explained: "It's just concentration." "Everyone will naturally enter a light state several times a day—think about it once you are planning the world when your friends share every detail of the vacation. Hypnosis is simply learning to require a useful way to focus your attention." Georgia has eliminated hypnosis's parable that makes people feel weird or scared from their patients' perspectives. She says she is usually sober and controlled. There are some exciting moments when to be told to tread on the size and see her target weight visually. "My creative mind must first imagine all clothes, jewelry, watches, and hairpins before beginning. Is anyone else doing this, or is it just me?" (No, not just you, Georgia!)

Ways to Lose Weight

Close your eyes. Imagine your food cravings. Imagine eating what good for you each day is. Imagine that hypnosis can assist you to reduce because the news is: indeed. Jean Fain, a psychotherapist at Harvard school of medicine, has provided you with ten sorts of hypnosis suggestions; please try it now. Once I tell people how I make a living by making a living (as a hypnotist and as a psychotherapist), they're going to ask: Does this work inevitably? My answer usually brightens their eyes between excitement and doubt.

Hypnosis is already available centuries before carbohydrate and calorie counting, but this ancient concentration technique has not been accepted wholeheartedly as an efficient weight-loss strategy. Until recently, there was little scientific evidence to support the legitimate claims of respected hypnosis therapists. Therefore, the massive commitment of their problem (stage hypnotists) didn't play any role.

Unless hypnosis causes you to or someone you recognize happy to shop for a replacement or smaller wardrobe, it's going to be hard to trust that this body-centric approach can help you control your diet.

So, take a glance at yourself. You do not need to bother finding some valuable lessons that hypnosis must teach you to reduce. Subsequent ten mini concepts include some weight loss methods that my weight management clients received during collective and individual hypnosis treatments.

The solution is inside. The hypnotherapist believes you've got everything you would need to succeed. You do not need other nutriment or the newest appetite suppressants. To reduce in weight is to believe your aptitude, just like riding a bicycle; at first, you will have a horrible experience as a first-timer, but you've got to keep practicing until you can automatically ride diligently. Losing weight seems to be beyond your scope, but it's just a matter of finding balance.

Believe it's to ascertain. People tend to realize what they think are often made; it even applies to hypnosis. The themes tricked them into thinking that they might hypnotize (for example, when the hypnotist suggested that they are angered, he turns on the hidden red bulb off) to prove the improved hypnotic response. The expectation of getting assistance is crucial.

If you imagine it, it'll come. Even as athletes steel themselves against the sport, visualizing victory can prepare you for the truth of success. Imagine a healthy diet each day, which will help you imagine the required steps to become a healthy dieter. Is it challenging to portray? Find an old photo of yourself, of moderate weight, and remember what you probably did differently at that time; imagine reviving those routines, or get advice visually from an older, smarter self which reaches the specified weight in the future.

Two strategies are better than one. In terms of weight loss and maintaining weight loss, the successful combination is hypnosis and cognitive-behavioral therapy (CBT), enhancing counterproductive thoughts and behaviors. Customers who have learned these two methods have lost twice their weight without falling into a dieter's disorder and regaining the trap. If you've ever written a food diary, you've already tried CBT. Before my clients learn hypnosis, they're going to track everything after every week or two. Every ethical hypnotherapist knows that raising awareness may be a crucial step towards lasting change.

Whether you wish or not, it's the way of life for the fattest person. There's no suggestion that there's enough power to exceed the survival instinct. It's the survival method; in the case of famine, we still program to survive the fittest. An honest example: a starving diet personal trainer who asked me to advise her to stop the jelly bear addiction. I attempted to elucidate that her body only believes that her life depends on chewy candies. She is not going to hand over the sweets until she has enough calories from more nutritious food. No, she insisted that she only needed one suggestion. I used to be unsurprised when she dropped out of the faculty.

Practice makes perfect. A Pilates session doesn't produce rubbing abs, and a hypnotic exercise doesn't improve diet. However, repeating 15 to twenty minutes of positive advice silently a day can change your eating habits, especially when combined with slow and natural breathing. It's the idea of any behavioral change plan.

Control craving. What if you'll get obviate cravings? Isolate them and send them out? Some weight loss hypnosis techniques can assist you to do that. For instance, you'll be asked to visually send your desires—like the case of a ship going on a bent sea. Recommendations also can assist you in reconstructing your desires and finding out how to manage them more effectively.

Looking forward to success. Expectations determine reality. Once we expect success, we naturally tend to require the required steps to realize success. Weight loss hypnosis can implant fruitful seeds in your brain, becoming a mighty unconscious power to help you stay in a healthy state.

Enthusiasm for practice. Negative factors often destroy weight loss. There are some foods that you "cannot" eat. Unhealthy food is "killing" you. Hypnosis therapy allows us to reimagine these suggestions with a more positive attitude—you won't lose yourself due to this; you're discarding what you do not need.

Able to relapse. We train to think that relapse is that shameful—the reason for abandoning. But hypnosis requires us to believe declines in several ways. Recurrence becomes a chance to see errors, learn from them, and steel oneself against temptation. Modify your behavior. A little step at a time can make big goals. Hypnosis therapy allows us to make small changes to realize larger goals. Suppose you reward yourself with sugary, high-calorie foods; through hypnosis, you'll choose healthier rewards.

Visualization success. Finally, hypnosis visualization may be a powerful motivation. The display allows you to "view" the results and explore how to cause you to feel. You'll also visualize your future self and tell yourself that you simply have everything you would need to succeed.

Congratulations, this is often a relapse. When customers find themselves over-indulging against their healthiest intentions, I congratulate them. Hypnosis treats regression as a chance, not a trivial matter. You'll be better prepared for the inevitable temptations in life if you'll learn from real or imagined relapses

Learn Self-hypnosis to Lead a Better Life

Wonder if you should practice hypnosis of yourself, or is it possible at all? Many people freak out when I mention they are supposed to learn the techniques of hypnosis, not even knowing what self-hypnosis is and how it can benefit their lives in several ways.

We are often witnesses to many serious problems in today 's fast lives, such as stress, time management and all kinds of mental disorders that people experience. We don't even know in most situations that we have some sort of problem in our mind, we just believe it's a temporary state of discomfort or nervousness that will pass by itself. Okay, they won't.

What about all the bad habits and personality traits we have developed over time? Smoking, over-eating, nail-biting, drinking, drug abuse, panic attacks, anxiety, social phobias, shyness, social life withdrawal, insomnia, lack of self-confidence, blushing, stuttering, binge eating, depression, anger, powerlessness ... And the list just keeps going on. The majority of people at any point in their lives will experience at least some of the above conditions.

That's why learning some techniques to clear up all the mess in your mind is essential to your overall well-being, and yesterday you should have started!

Your hands and teeth are typically washed many times a day, but how often do you clean your mind and soul? Have you already learned a method for doing it effectively?

There are many ways to relax and touch the subconscious mind to reprogram and alter it positively, and my personal opinion that one of the best ways to do this is to practice self-hypnosis. Once you master the technique, it won't take you more than 10-15 minutes a day to work on yourself to reach the ultimate goal, regardless of whether it's just to quit smoking or solve a lot of other issues.

It is not difficult to learn the essentials of self-hypnosis, and there is really no need to fear it.

The evidence for this is that over 500 million people are doing it every day around the world to get a better, healthier life.

Self-hypnosis is a state of mind, in which:

Extreme relaxation can happen

You pay special attention to the recommendations you want to bring into action

And helps you to acknowledge and not condemn the suggestions made.

Self-hypnosis helps you to program your subconscious directly with optimistic affirmations and helpful feedback and is a very successful way to alleviate and control stress and promotes deep relaxation in recovery.

Here we shall look at questions such as:

- When can I hypnosis myself practice?

- Where is self-hypnosis best practiced?

- How long am I supposed to practice self-hypnosis?

- Am I in a safe place to lay down or sit down?

- Will I need to close my eyes?

- Personal transition, what could I have expected?

- Is it possible to make the process some time easier?

When can I hypnosis myself practice?

Whenever you have a few minutes free from interruption, disruption or distraction, you can quite easily practice self-hypnosis. Nevertheless, you should never practice while driving, operating or working with any sort of machinery under any conditions whatsoever or while performing any other operation, task or process requiring your full and undivided attention.

Where is self-hypnosis best practiced?

Somewhere secure, clean, relaxed and quiet anywhere would be an ideal place for self-hypnosis practice. Usually indoors, though practicing self-hypnosis nearly anywhere is just as feasible.

If you ensure you can relax, feel relaxed and safe from as much external noise, discomfort or interference as possible, you can achieve more.

How long am I supposed to practice self-hypnosis?

Quality over quantity-as a guide 15 to 20 uninterrupted minutes of quality a day is more significant than 30 to 60 minutes of disturbance and disruption. Set aside a designated time when you are not going to be disturbed.

Keep in mind that all the time you invest in self-hypnosis will be reimbursed as you make a positive, life-affirming change about yourself. Train often as you become more professional you will definitely find that the time you need to train is will.

Am I in a safe place to lay down or sit down?

I achieve your self-hypnotic goal(s) by far more importantly being comfortable. Doing what you feel is most natural will work best and yield better results. Lying down to practice self-hypnosis might make drifting off to sleep too easy for you but if your ultimate goal is to fall to sleep then lying down would be fine.

Once again, many people find that sitting in a calm, supportive position with the assisted head provides the results they need.

Will I need to close my eyes?

Most people skilled in self-hypnosis can quickly and easily go into a trance with their eyes open, but most people feel more comfortable and would find it easier to start with eyes closed.

Personal transition, what could I have expected?

The outcomes you receive will be based solely on the suggestions you make during your self-hypnosis session. You can expect to make meaningful improvements to life, it's perfectly normal to expect the change that will improve your life. Transition is a normal part of our life; it happens to us and all those around us each and every day.

Is it possible to make the process some time easier?

Give yourself a suggestion that you will enter trance faster and easier next time during your self-hypnosis session. In a trance, an example may be: "I can easily return to this profoundly relaxed and concentrated state of consciousness whenever I want, simply by taking a few deep and calming breaths."

Self-Hypnosis - Practical Applications

How can you develop a self-disciplined cast iron and a strong will to succeed? With Self-hypnosis-

Convenient use

If for whatever reason, you do not already have good discipline, what could be the best way to acquire it quickly and effectively?

Every time you practice self-hypnosis, you'll experience a new burst of directional energy and commitment. When you observe what is happening every day in your life, you will constantly find that you are:

- Focus more on the personal and professional objectives

- Learn not to heed those times of self-doubt

- Break down procrastination, become a 'go-getter'

- Creating and sustaining a 'can do' mentality

- Achieve a greater sense of contentment and self-worth

How to practice Hypnosis of yourself

Find a place that is relaxed and quiet and sit down somewhere.

Relax your body by closing your eyes, and imagine relaxing waves running from your scalp down to your toes.

Feel the muscles relaxing in your body as relaxation waves wash them over.

Use suggestions to deepen a relaxing state. This can be as easy as saying: "I feel confident and comfortable with myself. I get more relaxed and comfortable with every step ..."

Use the affirmation(s) you want to install after you feel completely relaxed, you can mix these in with the suggestions for relaxation.

Self-hypnosis is an effective and practical technique for deep relaxation. It can be used with affirmations or without them, depending on what you want to achieve.

Find a comfortable and quiet place to sit down somewhere to use the technique. Think about it and plan, any comments you might want to make. Start with your eyes closed and your muscles relaxed. Using imagery is one good way to do this. Go ahead and use suggestions to relax even more. Using whatever affirmations, you have prepared when you feel really comfortable. Achieve hypnosis status for as long as you like.

CHAPTER 5:

Habits for Weight Loss

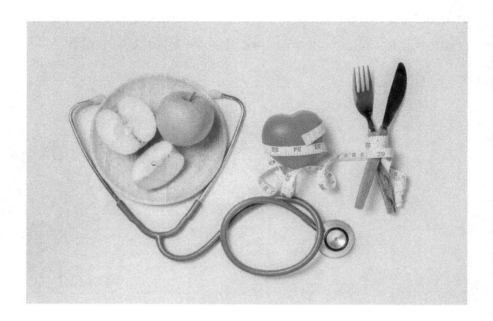

Take Things Slowly

Eating should not be treated as a race. Eat slowly. This just means that you should take your time in relishing and enjoying your food – it is a healthy thing! So, how long do you have to grind up the food in your mouth? Well, there is no specific time food should be chewed, but 18-25 bites are enough to enjoy the food mindfully.

This can be hard at first, mainly if you have been used to speed eating for an exceptionally long time. Why not try some new techniques like using chopsticks when you are accustomed to spoon and fork?

Or use your non-dominant hand when eating. These strategies can slow you down and improve your awareness.

Avoid Distractions

To make things simpler for you, just make it a habit of sitting down and staying away from distractions. The handful of nuts that you eat as you walk through the kitchen and the bunch of morning snacks you nibbled while standing in front of your fridge can be hard to recall.

According to researchers, people tend to eat more when they are doing other things too. You should, therefore, sit down and focus on your food to prevent mindless eating behaviors.

Savor Every Bite

Do not forget that eating mindfully is not only about enjoying the food you eat, but your health too, and without feeling guilty and uncomfortable. Relishing the sight, taste, and smell of your diet is utterly worth it. This can be so easy if you take things gradually and do not rush to perfection. Make small changes towards awareness until you are a fully mindful eater. So, eat slowly and savor the good food you are eating and the proper nutrition you are giving to your body.

Mind the Presentation

Regardless of how busy you are; it is a good idea to set the table – making sure it looks divine. A lovely set of utensils, placement, and napkin made of eco-friendly cloth material is a perfect reminder that you need to sit down and pay attention when you have your meals.

Plate Your Food

Serving yourself and portioning your food before you bring the plate to the table can help you to consume a modest amount, rather than putting a platter on the table from which to replenish continually. You can do this even with crackers, chips, nuts, and other snack foods. Keep yourself away from the temptation of eating straight from a bag of chips and different types of food. It is also helpful if you resize the bag or place the food in smaller containers so that you can stay aware of the amount of food you are eating. Having a bright idea of how much you have eaten will make you stop eating when you are full, or even sooner.

Always Choose Quality over Quantity

By trying to select smaller amounts of the most beautiful food within your means, you will end up enjoying and feeling satisfied without the chance of overeating. With this, it will be helpful if you spend time preparing your meals using quality and fresh ingredients. Cooking can be a pleasurable and relaxing experience if you only let yourself into it. On top of this, you can achieve the peace of mind that comes from knowing what is in the food you are eating.

Do Not Invite Your Thoughts and Emotions to Dinner

Just as there are many other factors that affect our sense of mindful eating, as well as the digestive system; it would come as no surprise that our thoughts and emotions play just as much of an important role.

It happens on the odd occasion that one comes home after a long and tiresome day and you feel somewhat "worked up," irritated and angry. This is when negative and even destructive thoughts creep in while you are having supper.

The best practice would be to avoid this altogether. Therefore, if you are feeling unhappy or angry in any way, go for a walk before supper, play with your children, or play with your family pet. But, whatever you do, take your mind off your negative emotions, before you attempt to have a meal.

Make a Good Meal Plan for Each Week

When you start the diet, it is advised to stick to the meal plan that comes with the diet. There should be a meal plan of 2 weeks or 4 weeks attached to the diet's guideline. Once you are familiar with the food list, prohibited ingredients, cooking techniques and how to go grocery shopping for your diet, it will be easier for you to twist and change things in the meal plan. Do not try to change the meal plan for the first 2 weeks. Stick to the meal plan they give you. If you try to change it right at the beginning, you may feel lost or feel terrified in the beginning. So, it is advised to try and introduce new recipes and ideas after you are 2 weeks into the diet.

Drink Lots of Water

Staying hydrated is the key to living a healthy life in general. It is not relevant for only diets, but in general we should always be drinking enough water to keep ourselves hydrated. Dehydration can bring forth many unwanted diseases. When you are dehydrated, you feel very dizzy, lightheaded, nauseous, and lethargic. You cannot focus on anything well. Urinary infection occurs, which triggers other health issues.

Being on a diet, the purpose of drinking water is to help you process the different food you are eating and to help digest it well. Water helps in proper digestion; it helps in extracting bad minerals from our body. Water also gives us a glow on the skin.

Never Skip Breakfast

It is essential to eat a full breakfast to keep yourself moving actively throughout the day. It gives you a great boost, good metabolism and your digestion starts properly functioning during the day. When you skip breakfast, everything sort of disrupts. Your day starts slow and soon you would feel restless. It is especially important to have a good meal at the beginning of your day in order to be productive for the rest of the day.

If you are terribly busy, try to have your breakfast on the go. Grab breakfast in a box or a mason jar and have it in the car or on the bus or whatever transport you are using to get to your work. You can also have your breakfast at a healthy restaurant where they serve food that is in sync with your diet.

Eat Protein

Protein is particularly good for the body. It helps your brain function better. Protein can come from both animal and non-animal products. So even if you are a vegetable or vegan, you can still enjoy your protein from plants. Soy, mushroom, legumes, and nuts are a few examples. Eating protein keeps you strong and healthy. Eating protein increases your brain function. On the other hand, if you do not eat enough protein for the day, your entire way would be wasted. You will not be able to focus on anything properly. You would feel dizzy and weak all through the day. If you are a vegetarian, or vegan you can enjoy avocado, coconut, almond, cashew, soy, and mushroom to get protein.

Eat Super Foods

Most people eat foods that do not necessarily affect them in the best way. Where some foods may enhance some people's energy levels, it may impact others more negatively. The important thing is to know your food. It may be a good idea to keep a food journal, and if you know that certain foods affect you negatively, one should try to avoid those foods and stick to healthier options. It is a fact that most people enjoy foods which they should probably not be eating. However, if you wish to eat mindfully and enhance your health and a general sense of wellbeing, then it would be best to eat foods that will precisely do that.

There are also various foods that are classified as superfoods. These would include your lean and purest sources of protein, such as free-range chicken, as well as a variety of fresh fruit, vegetable, and herbs.

Stop Multitasking While You Eat

Multitasking is defined as the simultaneous execution of more than one activity at one time. Though it is a skill that we should master, often it leads to unproductive activity. The development of our economy leads to a more hectic way of living. Most of us develop the habit of doing one thing while doing another. This is true even when it comes to eating.

Smaller Plates, Taller Glasses

This habit changer ties in a little bit with drinking more water; however, it is a bit different. People tend to fill up their plates with food, so the size of the plate matters. If you have a large plate, you are going to put more food on your plate but, if you have a smaller plate, you will have less food on your plate.

Stay Positive

The secret to succeeding in anything is being positive. When you start something new, always stay positive regarding it. You need to keep a positive mind, an open mind rather. You cannot be anxious, hasty, and restless in a diet. You need to keep calm and do everything that calms you down. Overthinking can lead to being bored and not interested in the diet very soon. The power of positivity is immense. It cannot be compared with anything else.

On the other hand, when you start something with a negative mindset, it eventually does not work out. You end up leaving it behind or failing at it because you had doubts right at the beginning. A doubtful mind cannot focus properly, and the best never comes out from a doubtful mind.

Eating mindlessly can cause anyone to eat way too much and this is what happens to most of us. The problem is that when people are eating, they are hardly thinking about what they are doing. Instead, their minds are on other things and this leads them not to be aware of how much they are eating.

Beware of the portions.

Many individuals eat approximately twice the average amount of meals consumed. Restaurants also deliver large servings, which will teach your mind to believe that the quantity of food the body requires is not beneficial to have hands-on the right serving proportions

Put the spoon down in between the bites.

It forces you to eat more gradually, which would be an easy calorie-cutting strategy. Whenever you take your time rather than snorting your meals, your body will naturally enroll the feeling of satiety that can take approximately 20 minutes to signal your brain. Plus, gradually eating will help the food to taste even better.

Gulp down water 24/7.

Although the body is basically a fairly smart tool, it can be vulnerable to slip-ups. "Sometimes, it is dehydration that triggers what you believe is a hunger pang. The" hunger "will lead you to snack because all your body requires would be some water.

Taking some time out to make lunch.

Not only can you save time by cooking your own lunch, but it can also make sure you exactly realize what you're putting in your body, so you get the correct foods. You're still less prone to miss lunch on busy days because you can only walk to the supermarket instead of trying to run out to purchase food. While missing those meals could help improve weight reduction, trying to deprive your body of regular meals will make you more likely to overeat it later.

Do not do anything else whilst you eat.

Focusing on food while there's stuff to do and viewing Instagram may be difficult, but munching away while you're disturbed will lead you to unintentionally indulge with more than you should. Disturbed food doesn't only create further intake at the time; it can also force you to consume further later in the day than is required.

Emphasize breakfasts.

"Eating a meal packed with healthy fiber and protein should keep you satiated, and will help you make healthier food decisions every day. Choose meals that are not carbohydrate explosions without something significant to hold you full, such as hash browns, warm cereal, and croissants, to maximize breakfast power. "Try poached eggs on the whole grain toast, simple Greek yogurt with a bowl of your preferred fruit, or a veggie-laden omelet.

Be clever when snacking.

If you're attempting to lose weight, snacking may be either your best friend or a potentially supportive, but undoubtedly manipulative saboteur. There's the problem of unknowingly getting in more than you thought, which you can remedy in a snap by pre-portioning the treats as per their portion sizes instead of only gnawing away at them willy-nilly. Another issue with snacking can arise if you eat without check throughout the day, rather than snacking mindfully. Check out the snacking habits for weight loss tips to make sure you are on the right path.

Sleep through adequate hours each night.

It may be tough to adhere to a healthy sleep schedule — especially while there are episodes of serial to catch up on — but having adequate rest is an effective way to promote weight loss. Sleeping helps maintain the hunger hormones leptin and ghrelin in control. Without an appropriate quantity, those hormones get unbalanced and may contribute to increased appetite.

Keep eating healthy as well on Sundays.

If you're infatuated with having eaten possibly the best Monday through Friday but consider weekends an unrestricted-for-all food, you might not see the weight loss you're hoping for.

If you add it all up, trying to eat poorly and not exercising Friday through Sunday tends to come out to 12 days off a month.

Instead of allowing weekdays to impact your habits, focus on achieving a positive lifestyle — with the occasional treat — that's feasible.

Concentrate upon small plates.

If you look at the same amount of food on a tiny plate vs. a big one, your eyes could tell you there's even more awesomeness on the smaller plate. Even though you don't consume enough, cutting down on the amount of plate area surrounding your food will drip your mind.

However, doing its opposite may trigger your appetite by forcing you to think you only ate a little bit.

Scale back on eating in family style.

When you dine with serving dishes full of extra help right in front of you, you can slip into refilling your plate carelessly even if you're not still hungry. Instead, if feasible, restrict the meal on the table about what you have to eat. This is not to conclude seconds are strictly prohibited — just review in and see if you're still starving prior to actually getting back to reach a little more.

In restaurants, the seat faced away from the buffet table.

Seeing more food in your sightline will drive you into food-coma territory, particularly if you're trying to maximize the benefit of your money. Instead of eating when thinking about what you can reward yourself with next, turn your attention to the other food, and concentrate on just embracing what's on your dish. If you'd like more food once you're finished, the buffet would still be there.

Place vegetables up on the plate.

One of the easiest strategies to fall into a healthier eating routine is by introducing foods to the diet rather than cutting them. Failing to consume all of the beloved snacks will go end up backfiring in a spree, whereas gradually raising your food consumption will only produce positive results. "Not only are veggies packed with essential nutrients to keep the body balanced and energized, but they also provide fiber to makes you lean. Beginning small to prevent vegetable burnout: add a cup of them just to at most one meal per day for a week and continue to integrate them into even more foods once you get accustomed to them.

Keep a diary of food.

If you practice any of these, but you don't see any significant weight reduction, it may seem like a complicated problem you really can't break. Keep a diet diary in any situation, such that you'll have a thorough and overall image of your behaviors. "It will help you identify places that are unique to both you and the habits that might use a little adjustment. Do the utmost and maintain control with the food and drink consumption for a whole week and check out and see whether you are unintentionally getting in a few additional calories that you should leave out and achieve the results you are seeking. Note, above all, that losing the weight always requires certain experimentation — but the idea is this is a long way you're practicing how to be healthy with the fitness, which really counts.

CHAPTER 6:

Benefits of Intuitive Eating

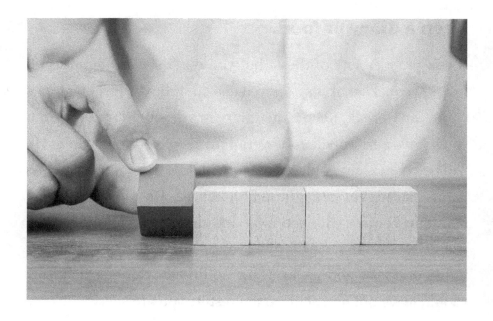

Intuitive eating is a non-diet approach, mind, and body approach to wellness and health. This approach doesn't encourage dieting but emphasizes taking note of the inner body and hunger cues. By trusting our bodies, intuitive healing renews our relationship with food.

Though it doesn't encourage dieting, it uses nutritional information to form healthy eating choices and habits. By this habit, we eat because we'd like to not because we've to, and dietary values are accepted disinterestedly. During this method, we rely more on our intuition. Food is employed to satisfy a requirement. Without the inner cue of hunger, no need for food. Those that want to flee the strain of dieting can appreciate this approach since it's useful and practical. There's no connection between emotions and food during this sort of eating.

Intuitive eating is not intended for weight reduction. Sadly, there might be dietitians, mentors, and different experts that sell intuitive eating as a diet, which runs counter to the thought altogether. The objective of intuitive eating is improving your association with food. This incorporates building more beneficial food practices and trying not to control the scale. That being stated, pretty much everyone experiencing the way toward figuring out how to be an intuitive eater needs to get thinner—else, they would as of now be intuitive eaters!

Intuitive eating enables your body to break the diet cycle and sink into its regular set point weight territory. This might be lower, higher, or a similar weight you are at present.

How Intuitive Eating Plays a Role in Healthy Living and Shopping Lifestyle:

Intuitive eating guides our lives inside and out. It creates such a lot of opportunity and straightforwardness by not stressing over what I will eat or when I will eat it. I stream with what my body guides me to eat, and when it guides me to it eat-and with that, it creates opportunity inside my relationship in my body and how I feel about myself. I am more advantageous and more adjusted than I have ever been in my body and I can say that I love my body and this vessel that I am carrying on with this life in. This move-in my association with my body, food and my general surroundings is an immediate consequence of my otherworldly voyage.

The most significant thing is to not stress over the 'right' or 'wrong' choice, and instead to distinguish how you are feeling and where in your body you think it-with the goal that you aren't eating to keep away from or conceal feelings. That way, your eating decisions are simpler to make since they are not enveloped with your passing feelings.

There is such a lot of opportunity and facilitate that shows up when you interface with and pursue your instinct. Shopping for food turns out to be, to a lesser degree a task or a problem and increasingly an action of happiness and articulation. To have the option to purchase what looks, sounds, and scents great (offers to the faculties) and to believe my instinct as far as what I will cook and create each day/week. It additionally makes the creation procedure progressively fun since you do not feel adhered to pursue a formula or dinner plan. Once more, there is an opportunity. Shopping for food is only an expansion of that and part of the creation procedure (where motivation comes in).

Indeed, there might, in any case, be times when you do not feel like shopping for food or preparing; however, in those minutes, you are not hung up on it. The dread of settling on an inappropriate choice or eating inappropriate food vanishes. Intuitive eating is not about control and dread; it is about the stream and following what feels better (from a space of instinct, not damage or self-hurt).

You are beginning the adventure of understanding what foods reverberate with your body, and what doesn't-interfaces with the act of enthusiastic mindfulness. On the off chance that we shut ourselves off from feeling our feelings, at that point, we are additionally closing our capacity to feel different sensations. Consider it like this-your body is sending you the flag of what feels better and what doesn't; however, you have unplugged the wire association between the inclination, and you are accepting and being informed of the disposition.

Having an essential comprehension of sustenance is a great spot to begin to start to teach oneself and acclimate oneself with specific establishments of pure sciences. From that point, it truly is an act of backing off and carrying your attention to how you feel previously, during and after eating. At whatever point you notice examples of side effects, you should investigate. What musings did you see, how could you feel, what was going on around then? A great deal of our food and eating practices/designs have been adapted and created quite a while prior and requires bringing our cognizance again into that space to develop progressive movements. The most significant piece of this procedure is to curry sympathy with you and practice non-judgment.

The diet culture is a finished square to instinct. It is established in dread and control-and expels the opportunity to interface with how you feel or what your body wants. The diet culture mirrors the longing to change and control the body, instead of helping it and work with it. It is tied in with stifling the body's direction framework (through control), which expels you further away from your instinct and the capacity to interface with your intuition through your body's informing structure. The greatest thing to perceive is that your body is profoundly insightful and realizes what to do-the more that you work with it and backing (and trust it)- the more joyful you will feel.

At whatever point we hop onto a pattern it is imperative to associate with what feels better (and to inquire as to whether this pattern genuinely impacts you or on the off chance that you are merely doing it since others are, and their outcomes entice you). A great spot to ground yourself in what your intuitive direction is, is to ask yourself "What feels useful for your spirit?"

The Health Benefits of Intuitive Eating

<u>There Is No Room for Stress:</u>

Studies have demonstrated that intuitive eaters not just appreciate a more lovely enthusiastic state than dieters, yet additionally experience enhancements in despair, nervousness, negative self-talk, and general mental prosperity when they change to eating intuitively.

The explanation behind this decrease in pressure may originate from the way that when you eat intuitively, you get the chance to concentrate more on making the most of your food as opposed to dissecting it. You additionally remove yourself from the outlook of, "I can't have that since I have to get thinner," or "I can't have carbs because I'm fat."

These sorts of responses to food put a heap of weight at the forefront of your thoughts and body, so it is no big surprise you feel better when you let them go!

Improvement in Digestion:

Two of the fundamental precepts of intuitive eating are to:

- Eat just when you are ravenous,

- Eat until you are fulfilled, not stuffed.

- Rehearsing both propensities can help improve your assimilation in various manners.

For one, eating just when you are genuinely hungry gives your stomach related framework time to discharge your stomach from your last supper. This may appear no major ordeal, and however, when you continue eating each couple of hours and not enabling your food to process, your framework can undoubtedly move toward becoming exhausted. Your stomach needs to consistently siphon out chemicals and acids to help digest your food, while your liver is ceaselessly being attempted to channel poisons and condensation fat.

Additionally, eating until you are full at each feast can shield your assimilation from running comfortably. You are basically "Backing up" your framework by pouring undigested food over half-processed food, which may make you experience acid reflux, stoppage, or any number of stomach related issues.

Rehearsing body mindfulness, eating just until you are fulfilled, and not eating between suppers except if you're eager gives your stomach related framework a rest with the goal that it's completely prepared to deal with your next dinner.

High Self-Esteem:

Notwithstanding improving eating examples and nervousness levels, contemplates have additionally demonstrated that rehearsing intuitive eating develops confidence.

For example, members in a single report experienced more acknowledgment of their bodies and less mental pain concerning their bodies. They were additionally ready to relinquish "Unfortunate weight control practices."

By improving your confidence, it is just typical that different parts of your life will improve too. At the point when you are concentrating less on not being "Sufficient," and more on tolerating yourself, you will generally encounter less nervousness and have an increasingly inspirational point of view. Thus, this can prompt many open doors at work and enhancements in your connections.

A Possibility to Aid Weight Loss:

Studies have likewise indicated that intuitive eaters have lower weight records (BMIs) than dieters. One of the significant purposes behind this could be because of the way that intuitive eating is anything, but difficult to adhere to (not at all like trend diets) which can prompt long haul weight reduction.

At the point when you eat intuitively, you additionally figure out how to regard the satiety flag that discloses to you when you are fulfilled, versus only eating for eating. This outcome is a natural, ideal calorie balance that could prompt weight reduction on the off chance that you have been overeating by disregarding yearning signs.

The way that intuitive eating lessens feelings of anxiety can likewise assume a job since a lot of the pressure hormone cortisol can cause fat addition.

A Decent Improvement In Body Awareness:

Monitoring your body and what it is motioning to you is critical with regards to keeping up your wellbeing. On the off chance that you listen intently, your body will offer you inconspicuous hints that something is not right, enabling you to give it what it needs before it turns into a significant issue.

Take, for instance, indications of supplement inadequacies. Numerous individuals are so separated from their bodies that they do not see unobtrusive signs of a supplement insufficiency, like an absence of vitality or shivering in their grasp and feet. When they do understand, the inadequacy has turned out to be dangerous to such an extent that they need to go to the specialist to get it dealt with.

Intuitive eating is tied in with connecting with your body's sign of craving and satiety. Be that as it may, when you start focusing on these signs, you will begin to be hyper-mindful of different signs your body is emitting. This will enable you to be in line with what you need consistently, so you can deal with it before it turns into an all-out issue.

CHAPTER 7:

Hypnotherapy for weight loss

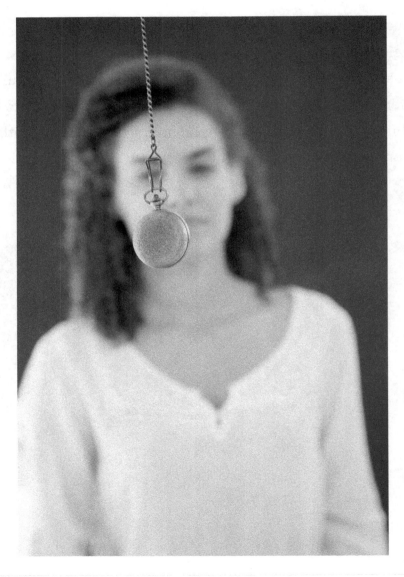

To put oneself in a state of hypnosis, or to make hypnosis with a practitioner, is to intentionally reproduce this state of consciousness with an objective that varies according to the framework in question (relaxation, care, personal development, etc.).

The hypnotic state is the reproduction of a natural and spontaneous state; everyone can have access to it, but not necessarily in the same way. While most individuals respond well to direct verbal suggestions, others will need an indirect approach to bring about the desired altered state of consciousness.

On the other hand, learning the method and its regular repetition allows everyone to be able to enter hypnosis with greater ease and speed: as with a sport, the more you exercise and the more you progress!

Does hypnotherapy work for weight loss?

Hypnosis can be more successful for those trying to lose weight than diet and exercise alone. The aim is to be able to manipulate the mind and alter behaviors like overeating. Nonetheless, it's always up for discussion just how powerful it can be.

An earlier, controlled trial examined the use of hypnotherapy in people with obstructive sleep apnea for weight loss. The research explored two different types of hypnotherapy and basic nutritional recommendations for weight loss and sleep apnea. Within three months, all 60 participants lost 2 to 3 percent of their body weight.

The hypnotherapy participant had shed, on average, an additional 8 pounds at the 18-month follow-up. While this additional loss was not significant, the researchers concluded that hypnotherapy justified more studies as a treatment for obesity. A weight-reduction study that involved hypnotherapy, primarily cognitive-behavioral therapy (CBT), found that this culminated in a slight drop in body weight relative to the placebo community. Researchers have hypothesized that although hypnotherapy can improve weight loss, there is not enough work to persuade them.

It's important to remember that there is not any evidence for weight reduction in favor of hypnosis alone. Most of what you'll learn in conjunction with food and exercise or treatment is in hypnotherapy.

Hypnotherapy Can Aid You to Change Developed Habits through the Power of Hypnosis

Crack the cycle of comfort eating by resolving the issue at the point that it is rooted in the unconscious mind. You can see some important improvements take place over the process of hypnotherapy treatment:

You're becoming more comfortable and your thinking is simpler

Holding the emotional and social needs apart will start to sound normal and therefore inevitably happen

You should search for more innovative ways to channel the thoughts and work with them

The appetite for healthier food will increase and it will significantly boost the diet

You will continue to feel more optimistic, more comfortable, and satisfied with your everyday life without a relentless cross.

Why Hypnotherapy for Losing Weight Can Help You

Have you ever wondered about food as if it were your friend? Have you ever thought that your family and friends are a priority? If you sincerely answer every one of these inquiries, you will come to learn that food is intended to be your companion. You would certainly regard it with greater respect when speaking about it in that manner. Since we just have one body and our health care bill worsens with time, we are most likely expected to take care of ourselves. The same refers to kicking unhealthy habits such as smoking, eating too much alcohol, likely taking mind-altering medications, and also other harmful effects such as sleep deprivation. Hypnosis is all about changing yourself, and you can eventually shift your attitude about diet, exercise, and unhealthy behavior if you will enter a place where you are concentrated on enhancing your health and are able to do so on a regular basis. It would become part of the routine to consume food that is good for your health. Having an ambitious target for yourself, such as completing 21 days of eating healthy, will inevitably lead to all those results if you continue to stick to self-hypnosis. You will build new routines and commonalities for twenty-one days of stability, which will hold you onboard long when you have met your targets for weight loss. Healthy eating after some time will not feel like a penalty, but more like a treat. You'll feel healthier by eating better, but also consuming less If you're like most individuals, you probably enjoy food and eating in general; that doesn't mean that you can't love your meals simply because you practice a diet and exercise schedule. Bearing in mind, though, that you have 3 meals per day, and probably snacks once or twice a day, you should be conscious that not that much food is needed for your body. If the measurement of your both hands clasped together in a fist is the size of your stomach, so where does the majority of the food you eat go? It gets stored as body fat, which is just what you don't like. Concentrate on feeding mindfully and listening to the body. You will also learn that consuming less really leaves you more comfortable. One of the biggest effects of hypnosis promotes your mentality about food and exercise. It changes your mood greatly. While certain individuals who participate in hypnosis use so to monitor their dietary patterns, the sedentary lives of most people are subject to a tone of adjustments. You are a human being, and you are supposed to run, search, and catch. You will rot away and die if you keep sitting all day and don't drive your body out of its comfort bubble.

The work of the hypnotherapist

Generally, the first session begins with an interview with the consultant in order to define his needs, and to determine the approach and methods to be used. This very first session is generally longer than the following and each technique is adapted to the client's needs. A typical session lasts 50 or 60 minutes. Most people start to see results after 4 meetings. Hypnosis is recognized as brief therapy. A dozen meetings are generally sufficient, at least for well-defined problems. In children, usually easier to hypnotize, changes are often seen after only 1 or 2 visits.

How to choose your hypnotherapist?

Don't just rely on word of mouth. It is useful to learn about the internet and to take the time to read the advice and information provided by the practitioner. These are important and allow you to get an idea of his style and approach. You can also call the practitioner to discuss your needs and expectations. It is essential to go to a professional with excellent training in psychotherapy or health, depending on the case to be treated. Ideally, he should know the mechanisms of the problem at hand, whatever it is (physical, psychological, relational, etc.). However, more than the techniques used by a given therapist,

Hypnotherapist, hypnotist, what differences?

The hypnotherapist is a specialist who uses hypnosis in order to treat and support his patient towards well-being, while the hypnotist designates an individual who knows how to bring about the state of hypnosis. While the former must have training and practice in the health sector, the latter is more active in the entertainment sector. Even though they both use hypnosis, the end goal and the context are completely different.

12 Week Hypnotherapy Program

The most effective product we found for reducing weight was a 12-week hypnotherapy program.

The program does take some commitment as each of the hypnosis recordings have been split right into twelve sessions, among which needs to be listened to daily.

Week 1

In the first week of the hypnotic course, you are provided with the foundations for your brand-new weight management regimen.

Along with setting a weight-loss target on your own, you are additionally skillfully guided to eliminate a lot of your self-imposed restricting ideas surrounding your capability to produce and maintain a healthy and balanced, non-fat, and fit body.

Week 2

In the second component of the course, you learn precisely how to determine your body's all-natural signals. If you are starving, your body lets you recognize it!

When you are full, your body allows you to know! You will learn just how to identify between a desire and what to consume.

When you additionally use hypnotherapy to get over this emotional belief of what to eat, you will make sure that your daily consumption of food is significantly minimized.

Week 3

Neuro-Linguistic Programming (NLP) is used to change your mental patterns and practices. NLP is a highly effective and scientifically confirmed collection of strategies made to create immediate behavioral changes.

When used along with hypnosis, NLP ensures that behavioral adjustment is rapid advertisement long-term.

Week 4

Making use of hypnotic sessions to direct your memory back to the primary source of your over-eating, then removes the causes leaving you without emotional consumption.

Week 5

In week five, you are emotionally conditioned to drink a lot of water. Because it loads you up, water is an excellent help in weight loss.

Water intake reduces cravings pangs. It also has terrific lots of health and wellness advantages and gets rid of contaminants from the body.

Week 6

In these sessions, you are conditioned to incorporate light, natural exercise right into your everyday regimen to enhance your metabolic rate and slim down faster.

Hypnotherapy can be a significant help in any weight-loss program and has been revealed to generate some incredible results very quickly. Weight loss through hypnosis is not a "magic tablet."

It becomes compelling when combined with a physical weight loss regimen or diet regimen and exercise program. Water is a fantastic help in weight loss since it fills you up.

Week 7

At this point in the training course, you are conditioned to begin eating more healthily.

Week 8

This is designed to help you raise your metabolic price by gaining straight access to your subconscious mind and changing the plan it holds for your body.

Although, as we stated earlier, many other hypnotic CDs try this method, it functions in this course because you have already been conditioned to take more workouts!

The hypnotic ideas used during this week will help you get even more out of your exercise regimen and hence burn fat quicker!

Week 9

As you move closer throughout the hypnotic weight loss course, you will surely make use of the Swish method to ensure that the brand-new practices you have discovered come to be irreversible.

Week 10

Currently, it's time to make use of your subconscious mind's power to help you burn much fatter. Through the effective hypnotic pointers, you can command your subconscious mind to consume more of the kept fat in your body.

The training course will actively transform your consuming habits and exercise level even more!

Week 11

This week deals with the essential issue of self-image! Ensuring you have a positive self-image and a healthy and balanced respect for your body will ensure you stay healthy and balanced and do not abuse your brand-new ability to drop weight!

Week 12

Week 12 coatings your program. You ought to currently be seeing major arise from the work you have previously done. You are provided with recommendations that enhance your new practices and maintain you motivated to maintain a healthy and balanced fit body.

Using hypnotherapy as a quick-fix option for your weight issues will not work! Using it as a tool to aid you in shedding weight might well be the difference between success and failure. If you absolutely and truthfully choose to shed weight and establish a healthy and balanced body, hypnosis is most definitely a way to make the essential modifications easy, long-term, and rapid.

The program is a behavioral-change system made to assist you to attain your perfect weight and make that adjustment irreversible. Because it alters your behavior and attitude to food and exercise, at the subconscious degree, once you end up the course, it just really feels all-natural for you to preserve your brand-new healthy and balanced overview and practices to consuming and workout!

CHAPTER 8:

How to stay motivated

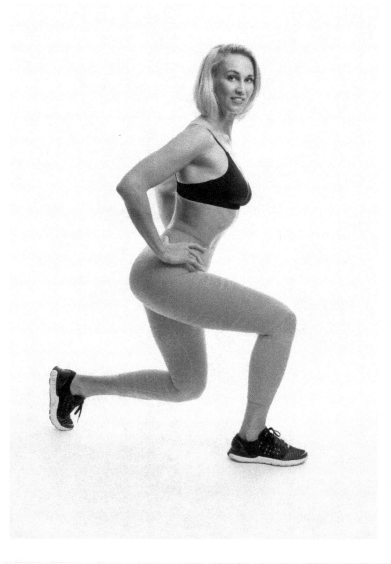

Motivation is one of the most powerful tools in creating permanent change. Your motivation is based on what you believe. And as you are probably aware, belief is scarcely based on your concrete reality. In essence, you believe things because of how you see them, feel them, hear them, smell them, and so forth. You can program your mind by taking feelings from one of your experiences and connecting those feelings to a different experience. Let us look at how you can remain motivated to lose weight:

Establish where you are now

You should take a full-length picture of yourself at present as a push mechanism from your current position. Two primary factors are relevant to health. One is whether you like the image you see in the mirror and the second is how you feel. Do you have the energy to do what you wish, and are you feeling strong enough?

Explore your reasons for wanting to lose weight. These are what will keep you going even when you don't feel like it.

Assess your eating habits and establish your reasons for overeating or indulging in the wrong foods.

It is assumed that you have the desire to get healthier and lose weight. Here, you state clearly and positively to yourself what you want, and then decide that you will accomplish it with persistence. Use the self-hypnosis routine explained above to drive this point into your subconscious mind.

Determine your motivation for the desired results, and how you will know when you've accomplished the goal. How will you feel, what you will see, and what are you likely to hear when you achieve your goal.

Devote the first session of self-hypnosis to making the ultimate decision about your weight. Note that you must never have any doubt in your mind about your challenge to lose weight.

Plan your meals every day. Weigh yourself frequently to monitor your progress as well. However, do not be paranoid about weighing yourself as this can actually negatively affect your progress.

Repeat to yourself every day that you are getting to your ideal weight, that you've developed new, sensible eating habits, and that you are no longer prone to temptation.

Think positively and provide positive affirmations in your self-induced hypnotic state.

Tweak Your Lifestyle

Every little thing counts. This is an important thing to note if you want to lose weight and slim down. Making a few changes in your regular daily activities can help you burn more calories.

Walk more

Use the stairs instead of the escalator or elevator if you're just going up or down a floor or two.

Park your car a mile away from your destination and walk the rest of the way. You can also walk briskly to burn more calories.

During your rest day, make it more active by taking your dog for a long walk in the park.

If you need to travel a few blocks, save gas and avoid traffic by walking. For greater distances, dust off that old bike and pedal your way to your destination.

Watch how and what you eat

A big breakfast kicks your body into hyper-metabolism mode so you should not skip the first meal of the day.

Brushing after a meal signals your brain that you've finished eating, making you crave less until your next scheduled meal.

If you need to get food from a restaurant, make your order to-go so you won't get tempted by their other offerings.

Plan your meals for the week, so you can count how many calories you are consuming in a day.

Make quick, healthy meals so you save time. There are thousands of recipes out there. Do some research?

Eat at a table, not in your car. Drive-thru food is almost always greasy and full of unhealthy carbohydrates.

Put more leaves, like arugula and alfalfa sprouts on your meals to give you more fiber and make you eat less.

Order the smallest meal size if you really need to eat fast food.

Start your meal with a vegetable salad. Dip the salad into the dressing instead of pouring it on.

For a midnight snack, munch on protein bars or just drink a glass of skim milk.

Eat before you go to the grocery to keep yourself from being tempted by food items that you don't really plan to buy.

Clean out your pantry by taking out food items that won't help you with your fitness goals.

The whole idea in the tweaks mentioned is that you should eat less and move more. You may be able to think of additional tweaks. List them down together with the ones found in this book.

Motivational Affirmation

Motivational affirmations are phrases, sentences, or even words that will enable you to stay positive, be focused, and be highly motivated. You need to choose these affirmations and use them on your daily basis. They are of great help as they will help you to meditate correctly on your weight loss. You can only reduce weight when you stay focused and positive. Being true to yourself and getting motivated every time will enable you to be able to control your weight. Even though these affirmations are numerous, you need to take a look at the ones I have detailed or illustrated the most common ones in the below paragraphs. It is good to note that, these affirmations, you can use each morning after just waking up. They will sincerely help you to jump-start your day on a much higher note. It is a challenge thrown at you that you better try this and see how your life will drastically change. Your mindset will shift, and you will only be thinking positively. You will only be staying focused on your life, and this will increase your esteem within and outside your external world. Below are some of the examples that you need to go through with much keenness.

You must embrace success. In every kind of situation or no matter the condition you are facing, tell yourself about success. You need to talk about being successful every morning. The word "you can't" should not appear in your mind. Everyone has excuses. Some excuses emerge from the fear of not trying. You need to stay focus and embrace the successful part of you. Don't get overwhelmed and overtaken by negative thinking about your success story. I challenge you to recite this affirmation every time you wake up. You will realize how important it is not only to your body but also in your external world. You need to feel unstoppable and fail to look at your excuses for not being successful. Negativity here is a BIG NO for you.

You must always be calm when faced with conflict. Conflicts are issues that always take you back to where you were. Conflict will automatically kill your daily morale leading to weak contributions of your abilities, especially within the organization and other sectors of life. You must try as quickly as possible to brush off annoyances easily. You must always agree with all sorts of disagreements so that the argument can end there. Tell yourself that you are more significant than what you are facing, and this should not drain you physically. Staying focused with a fit body and soul will make you lead a positive life.

At last, your weight will be highly controlled. You need to have that habit of doing this any time you are facing any conflict. It will only help you to stay positive and highly productive under your capacity. Reciting this affirmation every morning will be of great help. Try it as many as possible and help yourself to stay calm, relaxed, and comfortable.

You must choose to show love and gratitude every day. You need to know that life is always short and concentrating on negativity is not good. It won't go well with you. It will only derail your success. After all these, you must radiate elements of joy to yourself and have that love of your body. Showing all kinds of gratitude will enable you to lead a happy life. It will affect not only you but also the people around you. You must embrace this no matter what happens. Staying scorned and having negative thoughts only ages you as quickly as possible and leaves you with a body shape you never wanted. Be happy always and show love to the surrounding. You must try this and believe me, and you will have a change within the next few weeks.

You must be impressive to others. Staying positive in life is an excellent deal for yourself. Use anything under your disposal to impress those who are around you. You need to be positive in everything to be as positive as you can and never underrate yourself. No one sent a letter to be born in a certain way, so you need to accept yourself the way you are. It will enable you to stay focus and lead a real-life every day. You need to develop this habit of saying this affirmation to yourself as it is of great help. It will also help you to start your day with big morale and a notch higher.

You are free to develop your reality. Realities are things that are with us no matter what happens. Therefore, you must strive hard to create your reality. No one is supposed to create you one since you are in a better position with much knowledge about yourself. You must have a choice and choose wisely in every kind of situation you might get yourself herein. Remember, nothing should stand in between you and your happiness peak. That apex of goodness should be your cup of joy, and no one should prevent you from creating this form of reality for you. Choosing your reality every day will make you stay positive and entirely focused on life. Besides, it will be of great help as far as your body is concerned. Remember to note that your life ultimately depends on the realities within you. You can lie to people around you, but believe me, and you cannot lie to yourself. Therefore, it will be of great advice that you keep this affirmation as it will help you live and stay positive. In the end, this will automatically reflect on your body shape and image.

You need to shed off any unimportant attachment. Unimportant attachments are things that no longer have any effect on your life. These are things that will only let you down, thus derailing your life goals of achieving a mind-set full of happiness. Your future success depends heavily on this, and for you to get at that position, you will need to detach yourself from anything that might let you down. You must note that anything might also mean any person. We have people in our lives that always try very hard to put us down. These types of people are afraid of your success in life. They will try their best to pull you down, no matter how hard you try to embrace only positivity in your life. It is time to get yourself going and void them like the plague. Remember, you must live and not only live but choose a pleasant experience. It will only be possible if you manage to refuse anything or anyone that is holding you back. Since I have said this, it is now my wish that you may practice this affirmation and use it as your routine daily. Practice makes perfect, and you will only realize that when you train.

You are enough just as you are. You must release that demonic notion of having comparisons between you and others. For you to stay specific, you must have some success standards. After developing all these, set your own goals and ambitions. Your vision should relate to your mission in life. After all these, you can now judge yourself using the basis of your success. Those rules and regulations you created in your success standards should enable you to judge yourself accordingly. Just know you are just enough the way you were born. You are a complete soul, and no part of you is lacking. So never try to make a comparison with others. You should note that affirmation helps in the realization of worthiness. Within a short period, you will be able to control your body image. Also, it will be of a great deal as it helps you in achieving some of the personal goals in life and having a sound body is one of them.

You must be in a position to fulfill your purpose. The world should know your existence, and you must be ready to show your achievement. Showing your accomplished goals will need some positive deeds that lead to a successful life. On most occasions, people who trend are our trendsetters. They trend because of having done something positive or negative. They are then known all over the world. However, in this motivational affirmation, you need to focus on positive things. You need to be a trendsetter in showing the whole world what you are capable of offering. If you have been employed somewhere to sweep, you must clean until the country president cuts short his journey to congratulate you. Achieving your best is always one decisive way to be successful and lead a happy life free from stress and distress. Remember, this affirmation reminds you that no one has that power to stop you from doing or rather fulfilling your purpose in life. Sharing this thought every morning when you wake up will eventually get you somewhere. You must now stay focus and have this habit of telling yourself that no one can prevent you from achieving.

You must be results-oriented. In your daily life, you need to stay focus in life. Your primary focus should be on your results. It is through this that you will be able to realize your productivity.

To achieve this, you must be able to create some space for success. Get more success in your life. Avoid any derailing excuses that will only demean your reputation, thus lowering your success rate. Offer yourself these phrases every morning, and you will be in great joy for the rest of the day. You need not hold on to excuses for failing to achieve something. Be yourself and have the ability to struggle until you reach that success in life. It is through this that your mind will have settled, giving you peace of mind. Peace of mind will enable you to lead a stress-free experience. It will reflect in your body image.

Be in control of your won happiness. Happiness is an aspect of life that will initiate your feelings and moods towards a positive experience. It is like a gear geared towards your prosperous life. Staying positive here will be of great importance, and for you to realize this, you must take control of your happiness. Responsibility is a virtue and being responsible will make you bold enough to face all kinds of situations. Your joy is your key to success, and no one should tamper with it. Make happiness your priority and be responsible for it. You must let no one make you angry. Angriness will only induce you with emotional feelings that will eventually affect your life more so your body image. Having seen this, you must now be in an excellent position to embrace this affirmation. Take it as an opener to your morning and employ it entirely in your life.

CHAPTER 9:

The power of affirmations

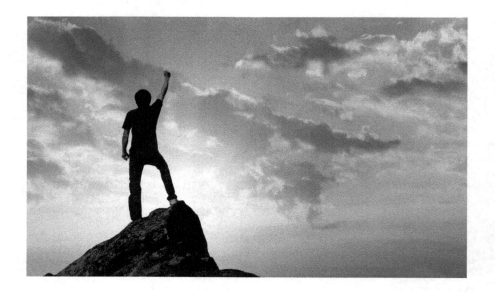

What Are Affirmations and the Way Do They Work?

Positive affirmations are positive statements describing a desired outcome, routine, or goal you wish to achieve. Repeating these positive statements often affects the subconscious mind deeply, and stimulates it into action, bringing into real life what you are parroting.

The act of mentally or loudly repeating the affirmations motivates the individual to repeat them, enhances confidence and inspiration, and creates incentives for change and success.

This act also programs the mind to act in accordance with repeated words, sparking the subconscious mind to work on one's behalf, making the factual claims come to fruition.

Affirmations are really helpful in creating healthy routines, achieving meaningful improvements in one's life, and attaining goals.

The affirmations help to lose weight, to become more centered, to learn more, to improve behaviors, and to fulfill goals.

They may be useful in athletics, industry, health-enhancing, bodybuilding, and many other fields.

These positive statements affect the body, the mind and one's feelings in a favorable way

It is very normal to repeat affirmations, but most individuals are not conscious of this. People often echo pessimistic, not constructive proclamations. This is known as negative self-talk.

When you tell yourself how miserable you are, how inadequate to learn, have not enough resources, or how tough life is, you reinforced pessimistic affirmations.

In this way, you generate more difficulties and many more issues because you focus on the troubles, and therefore increase them, rather than concentrating on the solutions.

Most people repeat negative words and statements in their minds about the unpleasant experiences and situations in life and thus create more unwanted situations.

Anytime you repeat something to yourself aloud, or in your thoughts, you're affirming something to yourself. We use affirmations consistently, whether we consciously know it or not. For instance, if you're on your weight loss journey and you repeat "I am never getting to lose the weight" to yourself daily, you're affirming to yourself that you only are never getting to succeed with weight loss. Likewise, if you're consistently saying, "I will always be fat" or "I am never getting to reach my goals," you're affirming those things to yourself, too.

When we use affirmations unintentionally, we frequently find ourselves using statements that will be hurtful and harmful to our psyche and our reality.

You might end up locking into becoming a mental bully toward yourself as you consistently repeat things to yourself that are unkind and even downright mean. As you are doing this, you affirm a lower sense of self-confidence, a scarcity of motivation, and a commitment to a body shape and wellness journey that you simply don't want to take care of.

Affirmations, whether positive or negative, conscious, or unconscious, are always creating or reinforcing the function of your brain and mindset.

Each time you repeat something to yourself, your subconscious hears it and strives to form a neighborhood of your reality. This fact is often because your subconscious is liable for creating your truth and your sense of identity.

It creates both around your affirmations since these are what you perceive as being your absolute truth; therefore, they create a "concrete" foundation for your reality and identity to rest on.

If you would like to vary these two aspects of yourself and your experience, you're getting to got to change what you're routinely repeating to yourself so that you're not creating a reality and identity rooted in negativity.

To vary your subconscious experience, you would like to consciously choose positive affirmations and repeat them continuingly to assist you in achieving the truth and identity that you only genuinely want.

This way, you're more likely to make an experience that reflects what you're trying to find, instead of an experience that reflects what your conscious and subconscious have automatically picked abreast of.

The key with affirmations is that you simply got to understand that your brain doesn't care if you're creating them intentionally or not.

It also doesn't care if you're creating healthy and positive ones or unhealthy and negative ones.

All your subconscious cares about is what's repeated thereto, and what you perceive as being your absolute truth.

It is up to you and your conscious mind to acknowledge that negative and unhealthy affirmations will hold you back, prevent you from experiencing positive experiences in life, and end in you feeling incapable and unmotivated.

Alternatively, consciously choosing healthy and positive affirmations will assist you with creating a healthier mindset and an identity that serves your wellbeing on a mental, physical, emotional, and spiritual level. From there, your responsibility is to repeat these affirmations to yourself until you think them consistently, and you start to ascertain them being reflected in your reality.

The only thing that is important when it comes to health and fitness is a balanced bodyweight. What decides your health is your weight! That's why, any time you go for a checkup, doctors always check your weight. The problem today is that people do not look at weight loss as a health problem anymore, instead of considering it as more of a looks problem, which is why they don't get anywhere. If they could only understand how important weight is to health, people would be more inspired to lose weight.

Your weight makes you who you really are. Whether you like it or not, you will be judged by it; this is just part of life. In fact, in America alone, over 65% of the population is either overweight or obese. That's two out of every three Americans. There are over 1 billion individuals worldwide that fall into this group! That's 1 in every 7 people around the world who have weight issues! It's no wonder healthcare is such a big issue.

So, you need to lose weight quickly and lose it right away, whether you're overweight or obese, but how are you going to lose weight the best way? The response to that is the biggest hidden weight loss mystery. The basic fact is that individuals DON'T know how to lose weight. In hopes that it will succeed, many will only try the old eat less and exercise more theory. Nonetheless, this mentality of weight loss is what ultimately keeps the world the same way with the same issues. People only do whatever the media and so-called experts tell them while doing the little operation. This is because there is no balance, which is why many struggle to lose weight!

The key to weight loss is balance. Every day, you need to eat the correct number of calories and exercise for the correct amount of time each week. For overall and long-term results, getting the balance is the best way! It's so important to understand because the secret of equilibrium can go to such endless depths.

However, you need to be well informed about it and its relationship with weight loss to make use of balance. You need to learn more about weight loss and all the elements of it. If you're serious about weight loss, then you can spend some of your time learning the secrets of weight loss. It's not going to be that hard if you know what there is to know about it.

If you want to really go further into weight loss, you're going to find there's so much more to it. Many factors have to be considered, including a good diet, weight, metabolism, and even the human body itself! In order to grasp weight loss entirely, there are so many things to remember.

You must first become educated about weight loss if you really want to commit to it. You need to get to the point where you will be able to spot it immediately if you make a mistake, without any support from experts or professionals. To succeed, you need to be totally alone.

Positive words are strong words that we repeat (either in our mind or out loud) to ourselves, and they are usually things we want to do. They are used to stimulate our inner thoughts and to affect our behavior and the progress we make. If you say them frequently with confidence and true conviction, then your subconscious mind will come to recognize them as genuine. Your new positive self-image will be improved, and you will be charged with positive energy. Your mindset, actions, and thoughts will shift and bring about a positive change until your mind begins to believe something is real. Positive remarks can be customized to any purpose you want to reach, including losing weight.

Try to use optimistic phrases that work for you and that you feel comfortable with. You have to repeat them regularly (at least 3-4 times a day) and with real certainty in order for them to work. Repeat them when you wake up in the morning and the last thing before you go to bed. Saying them out loud can be very motivational if you can get time alone. Write down your optimistic affirmations on a card and bring them around with you for an immediate boost at any time. You might also be able to post them on your fridge, a brilliant way to make you think twice about unhealthy snacks.

How's your loss of weight going? Are you losing the weight you thought you were going to lose? The expectations we set for losing weight often do not necessarily align with the actual act of losing weight. It can be really tempting to feel like it's pointless at times such as this, to just forget it and give up, then go back to the old way of eating.

In addition to keeping, you on track with your weight loss goals, optimistic words can be incredibly helpful by inspiring you to stay on this healthy track every day.

Affirmations and visualizations are tools that are used to accomplish almost anything in life, and there is no exception when it comes to weight loss. If that is so, why do so many people insist that statements don't work?

They need to be carried out properly in order for them to work. Some individuals feel that they can master a specific subject simply by seeking knowledge here and there. Quite often, in order to achieve success, a mastery of the subject is necessary.

The mediocre life that individuals build for themselves because of their negative thinking is a clear example of statements at work. Poor thinking plays a part in daily comments.

Note, it's not easy to do. Negative thinking is a custom, and it takes a deliberate, persistent effort to break a habit.

How to Use Affirmations and Visualizations for Successful Weight

Rule 1: never use phrases that are negative. Affirmations are directed towards the subconscious mind, and negative phrases are not defined by the subconscious mind. For instance, if you say "I am no longer overweight", the subconscious mind focuses on the "overweight" aspect and ensures that you stay overweight because it sees it as something you want.

Rule 2: using the claims only in the present tense. Do not say, "With this program, I will lose weight"; instead say, "I weigh 120 pounds right now" (if your target weight is 120 pounds).

Rule 3: be insistent. Don't give up ever. Everything you have now in your life is because of years of poor thinking. It will take some time before you begin to see good things about your life, but often you will be shocked by how easily things can change.

What keeps you from reaching your weight loss target? There may be several causes and explanations, such as medicine or disease, to blame for difficulty losing unnecessary pounds.

A hormonal imbalance can interfere with weight gain fluctuations. Emotional tension and adverse thoughts can dampen your spirits and send conflicting messages to your body. Just like your goals, a negative body image and attitude may also cause your body to respond.

Using helpful weight loss tips and motivation will set you on a healthy path, while melting fat cells to balance your body and mind.

Learning Affirmations is an Essential Step to a Slimmer You.

It could be said that there are literally dozens of proven and effective ways of programming your subconscious mind for weight loss hypnosis. However, out of all the hypnosis for weight loss techniques, none have the lasting power and motivating effect of positive affirmations. Why? Because it's a basic skill for lifelong success as your new slimmer self, well worth the time it takes to learn the skill, including how to write and use your affirmations, how to integrate them into your daily routine, and how to add them to your regular exercise. This article will explain how to use affirmations with hypnosis for weight loss.

It can take months for some clients to fully learn hypnosis for weight loss. I spent four weeks with Colin "under my wing". He studied some of the most effective personal enhancement techniques, and he studied almost all the tight-lipped secrets that weight loss hypnosis has to offer. However, once he began using three basic sentences, each day in three different settings, that was when he realized the improvements had taken place.

A basic formula for using affirmations and weight loss hypnosis is available. On an index card, you write down each and every one of your optimistic affirmations. Each day, you can take out a new card and re-affirm your statement. You can only start up again when you get to the end of the cards. You could have as few as three cards, or one for every day of the year. It comes down to whatever works for you best. The following are some examples of affirmations.

When it comes to affirmations, everyone is special, but here are the top three that I found with Colin. When you practice hypnosis for weight loss, you will find that you have your own favorites. "Day by day, I am getting slimmer and slimmer in every way." This is an old affirmation that has been around for years and has a compounding impact on the subconscious mind when properly repeated. "I am happy, safe, prosperous, and smart" and "I now have everything I need for permanent weight loss". Use these three affirmations as a start, and you can build ones that work for you with practice. Use them as follows.

In different settings, you may want to use these optimistic affirmations at least three times per day, including when you work out and before you go to sleep at night. You could even incorporate them into your morning walk to work. One instance is to say something when you work out, like "I have a fantastic body" and "I love my body". You are programming yourself with optimistic thinking, good emotions, and new habits that will affect you, even though you don't believe that this is valid. These new affirmations will soon become your normal way of thinking and repeating them over and over again will create a condition of self-fulfillment for you. You set yourself up to win.

In order to make your change last, it will take some engagement and constant effort on your part. So, make sure to learn and use these sample affirmations and produce your own weight loss script hypnosis. Do the exercises and compose and add your own affirmations that relate to you into your everyday life. The drug has been prescribed to you, and now it's your turn to take it.

How Do I Pick and Use Affirmations for Weight Loss?

Choosing affirmations for your weight loss journey requires you first to understand what it's that you are merely trying to find, and what sorts of positive thoughts are getting to assist you in getting there. You'll start by identifying what your dream is, what you would like your ideal body to seem and desire, and the way you would like to feel as you achieve your thought of losing weight. Once you've got identified what your idea is, you would like to spot what current beliefs you've got around the hope that you simply are meaning to achieve.

For example, if you would like to lose 25 pounds so that you'll have a healthier weight, but you think that it'll be incredibly hard to lose that weight, then you recognize that your current beliefs are that losing weight is tough. You would like to spot every single opinion surrounding your weight loss goals and understand which of them are negative or are limiting and preventing you from achieving your goal of losing weight.

After you've got identified which of your beliefs are negative and unhelpful, you'll choose affirmations that are getting to assist you in changing your beliefs. Typically, you would like to settle on a statement that's getting to help you completely change that belief within the other way.

For example, if you think that "losing weight is tough," then your new affirmation might be "I lose the load effortlessly." Albeit you are doing not believe this further affirmation immediately, the goal is to repeat it to yourself enough that it becomes a neighborhood of your identity and, inevitably, your reality. This way, you're anchoring in your hypnosis sessions, and you're effectively rewiring your brain in between sessions, too.

As you employ affirmations to assist you achieve weight loss, I encourage you to try to so in a way that's intuitive to your experience.

There are no right or wrong thanks to approaching affirmations, as long as you're using them daily. Once you are feeling yourself effortlessly believing in a statement, you'll start incorporating new affirmations into your routine so that you'll still use your affirmations to enhance your wellbeing overall. Ideally, you ought to always be using positive affirmations even after you've got seen the changes you desire, as statements are an exquisite thanks to naturally helping maintain your mental, emotional, and physical wellbeing.

What Should I Do with My Affirmations?

After you've got chosen what affirmations you would like to use and which of them are getting to feel best for you, you would like to understand what to try with them! The only thanks to using your affirmations are to select 1-2 statements and repeat them to yourself daily. You'll repeat them anytime you are feeling the necessity to re-affirm something to yourself; otherwise, you can repeat them continually, albeit they are doing not seem entirely relevant within the moment.

The keys to making sure that you simply are always repeating them to yourself so that you're more likely to possess success in rewiring your brain and achieving the new, healthier, and simpler beliefs that you got to improve the standard of your life.

In addition to repeating your affirmations to yourself, you'll also use them in many other ways. A method that folks like using statements are by writing them down.

You can write your affirmations down on little notes and leave them around your house; otherwise, you can make a ritual out of writing your statements down a particular number of times per day during a journal so that you're ready to work them into your day routinely. Some people also will meditate on their affirmations, meaning that they essentially meditate then repeat the affirmations to themselves over and over during a meditative state.

If repeating your affirmation to yourself sort of a mantra is just too challenging, you'll also say your chosen affirmations to yourself on a voice recording track then repeat them to yourself on loop while you meditate.

Other people will create recordings of themselves repeating several affirmations into their voice recorder then taking note of them on loop. At the same time, they compute, eat, drive to figure, or otherwise engage in an activity where affirmations could be useful.

If you want to form your affirmations productive and obtain the foremost out of them, you would like to seek out how to bombard your brain with this new information necessarily. The more effectively you'll do that, the more your subconscious mind goes to select abreast of it and still reinforce your new neural pathways with these new affirmations. Through that, you'll end up effortlessly and naturally believing within the new statements that you simply have chosen for yourself.

How Are Affirmations Going to Help Me Lose Weight?

Affirmations are getting to assist you in reducing during a few alternative ways. First and foremost, and doubtless most blatant, is that the indisputable fact that statements are arriving to help you get within the mindset of weight loss.

To put it simply: you can't sit around believing nothing goes to figure and expect things to think for you. You would like to be ready to cultivate a motivated mindset that permits you to make success. If you're unable to believe that it'll come true: trust that it'll not come true.

As your mindset improves, your subconscious is getting to start changing other things within your body, too.

For example, instead of creating desires and cravings for things that aren't healthy for you, your body will begin to make desires and cravings for items that are healthy for you. It'll also stop creating inner conflict around making the proper choices and taking care of yourself. You'll even end up falling crazy together with your new diet and your new exercise routine.

You will also likely end up naturally leaning toward behaviors and habits that are healthier for you without having to undertake so hard to make those habits. In many cases, you would possibly create practices that are healthy for you without even realizing that you simply are creating those habits.

Rather than having to consciously become conscious of the necessity for habits, then fixing the work to make them, your body and mind will naturally begin to acknowledge the need for better practices and can create those habits usually also.

Some studies have also suggested that using affirmations will help your brain and subconscious govern your body differently, too. For instance, you'll be ready to improve your body's ability to digest things and manage your weight naturally by using affirmations and hypnosis. In doing so, you'll be prepared to subconsciously adjust which hormones, chemicals, and enzymes are created within your body to assist with things like digestive functions, energy creation, and other weight- and health-related concerns that you may have.

You can use these affirmations as there; otherwise, you can adjust them to match what you would like for your belief system. If you are doing rewrite them, confirm that you simply are creating ones that directly reflect what you would like to listen to so that you'll change your beliefs to ones that are more supportive and less limiting.

Words work to build or demolish in both ways. It is the manner we utilize them that decides how they can produce positive or negative outcomes.

Positive affirmations to help you get started

- I'm grateful that I woke up today. Thank you for making me happy today.

- Today is a very good day. I meet nice and helpful people, whom I treat kindly.

- Every new day is for me. I live to make myself feel good. Today I just pick good thoughts for myself.

- Something wonderful is happening to me today.

- I feel good.

- I am calm, energetic, and cheerful.

- My organs are healthy.

- I am satisfied and balanced.

- I live in peace and understanding with everyone.

- I listen to others with patience.

- In every situation, I find the good.

- I accept and respect myself and my fellow human beings.

- I trust myself; I trust my inner wisdom.

- Do you often scold yourself? Then repeat the following affirmations frequently:

- I forgive myself.

- I'm good to myself.

- I motivate myself over and over again.

- I'm doing my job well.

- I care about myself.

- I am doing my best.

- I am proud of myself for my achievements.

- I am aware that sometimes I have to pamper my soul.

- I remember that I did a great job this week.

- I deserved this small piece of candy.

- I let go of the feeling of guilt.

- I release the blame.

- Everyone is imperfect. I accept that I am too.

- If you feel pain when you choose to avoid delicious food, you need to motivate yourself with affirmations:

- I am motivated and persistent.

- I control my life and my weight.

- I'm ready to change my life.

- Changes make me feel better.

- I follow my diet with joy and cheerfulness.

- I am aware of my amazing capacities.

- I am grateful for my opportunities.

- Today I'm excited to start a new diet.

- I always keep in mind my goals.

- I imagine myself as slim and beautiful.

- Today I am happy to have the opportunity to do what I have long been postponing.

- I possess the energy and will to go through my diet.

- I prefer to lose weight instead of wasting time on momentary pleasures.

- Here you can find affirmations that help you to change serious convictions and blockages:

- I see my progress every day.

- I listen to my body's messages.

- I'm taking care of my health.

- I eat healthy food.

- I love who I am.

- I love how life supports me.

- A good parking space, coffee, conversation. It's all for me today.

- It feels good to be awake because I can live in peace, health, love.

- I'm grateful that I woke up. I take a deep breath of peace and tranquillity.

- I love my body. I love being served by me.

- I eat by tasting every flavor of the food.

- I am aware of the benefits of healthy food.

- I enjoy eating healthy food and being fitter every day.

- I feel energetic because I eat well.

- Many people are struggling with being overweight because they don't move enough. The very root of this issue can be a refusal to do exercises due to negative biases in our minds.

- We can overcome these beliefs by repeating the following affirmations:

- I like moving because it helps my body burn fat.

- Each time I exercise, I am getting closer to having a beautiful, tight shapely body.

- It's a very uplifting feeling of being able to climb up to 100 steps without stopping.

- It's easier to have an excellent quality of life if I move.

- I like the feeling of returning to my home tired but happy after a long winter walk.

- Physical exercises help me have a longer life.

- I am proud to have better fitness and agility.

- I feel happier thanks to the happiness hormone produced by exercise.

- I feel full thanks to the enzymes that produce a sense of fullness during physical exercises.

- I am aware even after exercise, my muscles continue to burn fat, and so I lose weight while resting.

- I feel more energetic after exercise.

- My goal is to lose weight. Therefore I exercise.

- I am motivated to exercise every day.

- I lose weight while I exercise.

- Now, I am going to give you a list of generic affirmations that you can build in your program:

- I'm glad I'm who I am.

- Today, I read articles and watch movies that make me feel positive about my diet progress.

- I love it when I'm happy.

- I take a deep breath and exhale my fears.

- Today I do not want to prove my truth, but I want to be happy.

- I am strong and healthy. I'm fine, and I'm getting better.

- I am happy today because whatever I do, I find joy in it.

- I pay attention to what I can become.

- I love myself and am helpful to others.

- I accept what I cannot change.

- I am happy that I can eat healthy food.

- I am happy that I have been changing my life with my new healthy lifestyle.

- Today I do not compare myself to others.

- I accept and support who I am and turn to me with love.

- Today I can do anything for my improvement.

- I'm fine. I'm happy for life. I love who I am. I'm strong and confident.

- I am calm and satisfied.

- Today is perfect for me to exercise and to be healthy.

- I have decided to lose weight, and I am strong enough to follow my will.

- I love myself, so I want to lose weight.

- I am proud of myself because I follow my diet program.

- I see how much stronger I am.

- I know that I can do it.

- It is not my past, but my present that defines me.

- I am grateful for my life.

- I am grateful for my body because it collaborates well with me.

- Eating healthy foods supports me in getting the best nutrients I need to be in the best shape.

- I eat only healthy foods, and I avoid processed foods.

- I can achieve my weight loss goals.

- All cells in my body are fit and healthy, and so am I.

- I enjoy staying healthy and sustaining my ideal weight.

- I feel that my body is losing weight right now.

- I care about my body by exercising every day.

CHAPTER 10:

Increases your self-esteem every day

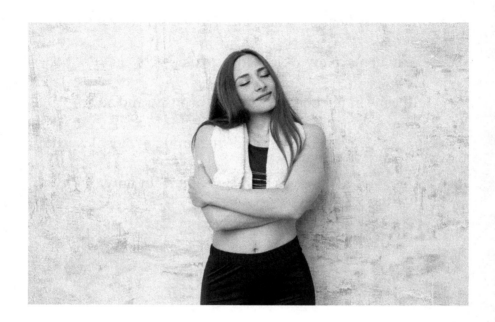

There's Self-Esteem, Then There's Confidence

You might be thinking that self-esteem and self-confidence are the same things--and many people do use those terms interchangeably--but there is a significant difference between the two. Self-esteem refers to how you value yourself. This is often based on social norms, and you frequently measure yourself in comparison to other people. For example, you might think, "I'm as intelligent and attractive as the next guy. Sure, I'm not a supermodel, but I'm not chopped liver either." Or, you might think, "I wish I were as witty as she is. I can't think of things to say as fast as most people can." Both of these statements reflect a valuation of yourself in comparison to other people.

If you have high self-esteem, you are comfortable in your skin. You're happy with who you are, regardless of how you might measure up to the next person. You can recognize and appreciate the gifts that other people might have, but this is important--you also acknowledge your contributions. You know that the offerings of other people do not detract from those of your own. You understand that you don't have to have the same gifts that everyone else has.

If you have low self-esteem, on the other hand, you will continuously not measure up, which can lead to depression and a sense of hopelessness. It can cause you not even to try because you think you will never succeed. You will also likely be submissive to other people's wishes because you don't believe you can lead the way, even if we're talking about your own life. Additionally, you'll often find yourself feeling guilty as if you have done something wrong when, in fact, you've done nothing to be guilty about. You might think you have to prove you're as good as someone else, and for that reason, you likely will set an unrealistically high standard for perfection. That sets you up for failure, which reinforces the low opinion you already have of yourself. It's a vicious cycle. But you might be thinking that you do have confidence in your ability to get things done. Ah, but confidence is a horse of a different color.

Self-confidence is how we view our ability to do something, like overcome an obstacle or improve a skill. It's really about how you perceive your ability to get the job done. While it is true that completing tasks successfully can increase your self-confidence, and that can, in turn, increase your self-esteem, it is also possible that you can have high confidence and low self-esteem. You can believe that you can get the job done and simultaneously think you're not the right person.

On the other hand, you can have high self-esteem and low self-confidence. You can value yourself as a person but question your ability to do the job. This might be exemplified by people you know with high self-esteem who are extremely competent at a particular task (or even many tasks), but who are continually questioning their work. They double and triple check themselves with every job they do. It's not that they think they're not intelligent enough to do the job, but they question their ability to get it done correctly. They always fear they will make a mistake. This is low self-confidence in action.

On the other end of the spectrum, people with high self-confidence can easily cross the line into arrogance. We tend to admire confident people, but what makes them sure is that they don't feel the need to advertise their skills. They know they have done the job well or have a particular talent, and they don't have to show off those skills to prove themselves. When people feel the need to flaunt their abilities, this is referred to as arrogance. In reality, it's another type of confidence, a false bravado that people project to cover what is likely their low self-esteem. These are the loud, opinionated, and often abrasive people in the presentation of their views. If someone feels the need to pander for adoration or is continuously looking to demonstrate they are the most knowledgeable or most capable individual, it likely indicates they secretly have a low opinion of themselves and seek external approval to prop up their self-image.

At this point, you might also be wondering about humility. Isn't being humble a good thing? Humility is defined as having a modest view of one's importance. But this doesn't mean exactly what it sounds like. It is not encouraging low self-esteem. Instead, there is a difference between how you value yourself as a person and how you view your contributions in life. For example, you can know you are the right person and that you contributed in a meaningful way to the successful completion of a project, but at the same time, you can know that it was a team effort that got the job done. You can also understand that the completion of the project is more important than any one person's contribution alone.

To sum it up, self-esteem is the value you place on yourself. Self-confidence is the view you have of your ability to get something done, and humility knows that, while you know you are valuable and capable, there are more important things than your accomplishments. Arrogance is when you feel the need to flaunt your abilities or achievements, and it often masks low self-esteem. But how do these things form? When do we develop our image of ourselves and our belief, or lack thereof, in our abilities?

The Impact of Social Media on Self-Esteem and Confidence

One of the problems with social media is that people tend to share only their highlights, which creates an image of constant happiness that might not reflect reality. It creates an unrealistic appearance with which you might be comparing yourself. It appears all your 'friends' are always enjoying life and experiencing success, and you feel like you're not measuring up.

But that's not reality. What you're not seeing is the behind the scenes struggles that they also go through as they face numerous challenges. They post that they got a new job, and you think, "Wow! How easy that was for them, and now they're off on a new, exciting adventure." However, what they didn't post were the numerous applications and perhaps some failed job interviews that came before they finally got the new job. You don't see the self-doubt they experienced about whether they would be able to find a new job. Also, it might not just be your friends' profiles that depress you. You might become depressed by your profile if you realize that your posting is an illusion. You might think you're not living up to your own best self.

Does this mean you have to stop using social media? Maybe! It would be best if you took whatever means are necessary to prioritize building up your self-esteem and confidence. Perhaps it doesn't mean you have to stop using social media but consider taking a break from it while you focus on yourself if you feel it is holding you back. Whatever you decide to do, you need to realize that what you see on social media is the best face put forward by your many friends. It's like pictures in a photo album; you don't see the sad moments or the depressing and challenging times. You see the happy times, the successes, and the smiles. But, it's just a moment in someone's life, and it's usually just the best moments that they take a picture of, and then post on social media. That doesn't mean they don't have bad moments too--they're just not posting those in the same way you are likely not posting your fears, anxieties, and difficulties in life. As with your 'physical' friends, you should seek out positive virtual friends and get rid of any virtual friends trying to tear you down. Virtual bullying can be even more damaging than what happens on the school playground since you can at least escape the playground. Be careful about who you "friend" --make sure they're someone who will appreciate you! Remember, all the rules of building your self-esteem and self-confidence apply to the virtual realm as well as the physical.

Managing the Media Impact on Self-Esteem for Healthy and Sustainable Weight Loss

What does your body resemble? The odds are that you have at any rate a couple of flaws that stress you and keep you from tolerating and cherishing your body.

As indicated by a 2014 report, almost 10 million ladies in the UK experience uneasiness and sorrow in light of their looks. One in every four ladies has avoided getting a charge out of a personal connection on account of her appearance. Almost 25 percent of the ladies examined detailed that stresses regarding appearance have kept them from seeking after work.

What's considerably more problematic - 36 percent of the ladies addressed said that they don't practice as a result of stresses over appearance and being taunted at the exercise center.

Media set inconceivable magnificence and wellness principles. By far most ladies would never draw near to those unreachable pictures of flawlessness.

Unimaginable self-perception depiction is additionally holding up the traffic of effective weight reduction by influencing self-discernment and fearlessness.

The Media Influence on Body Image

Media have sway on all ladies - from youthful and naive adolescents to senior women. One thing is sure - we don't appear as though big names and the exceptionally controlled pictures cause individuals to feel totally lacking in their skin.

Magazines, films, music clasps and sites all present unreasonable flawlessness. Obviously, a great deal of this flawlessness originates from picture handling, yet the photos are amazingly incredible and powerful.

Being fit and solid is adjusted to being thin, a condition that is unsafe yet that an ever-increasing number of individuals are beginning to grasp.

Positive Body Image for Successful Weight Loss

Effective and reasonable weight reduction ought to be about wellbeing instead of unreachable excellence beliefs. It requires a difference in attitude, which can be especially hard to achieve. Contrasting ourselves with others is an ordinary piece of human instinct and breaking out of the awful media cycle requires cognizant exertion and quality.

Investigate you - what number of models do you see strolling around? Customary ladies have bends, cellulite, stretch imprints, dull spots and different flaws. It's urgent to comprehend that you're contrasting yourself with something that doesn't exist.

Affirmations for Self-Esteem

When it involves body image, self-esteem is vital. Low self-esteem is often both the explanation for an undesirable body image and, therefore, the results of one. If you are unhappy with how you look and feel, it might be because you lack the vanity to form a change; otherwise, you may feel that way due to how your health is within the times.

Either way, boosting your self-esteem can now help keep you committed to your wellness goals and may improve your ability to foster a body shape and level of health that feels more desirable for you.

- I deserve a happy, healthy life and body.

- I'm a singular individual.

- Life is fun and rewarding.

- I need to have a body that helps me explore everything that life has got to offer.

- I select to be happy and healthy immediately. I like my life.

- I select to possess a pleasant experience.

- I really like and accept myself as I'm.

- I'm thriving now and forever.

- Every day I take a step toward becoming my best self.

- I need to love my body.

CHAPTER 11:

How to Use Meditation and Affirmations to Lose Weight

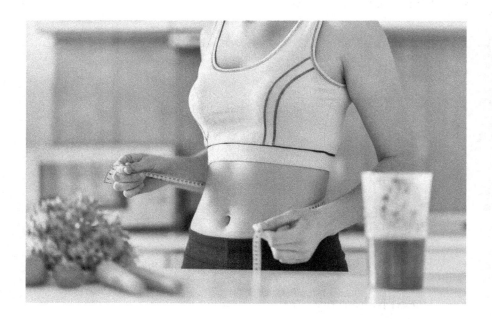

People always associate bodyweight genes or external factors like, eating habits, available food at one's disposal, or emotional stress. People do try to escape the fact that they are responsible for their eating choices and the quantity of the food they eat. This makes it easy to go back to our original poor eating habits even after we have started meditation. However, through meditation, we get to understand our role and contribution to our own journey to weight loss. Changing one's eating habits and patterns is not an easy step and requires a lot of patience, motivation, and focus. Always surround yourself with people who can motivate you to make healthier choices. We need not blame our genes but try to work on making better health choices.

Helpful Tips for Food and Meditation

Go slow with your meals, put more emphasis on chewing very slowly, and know the taste of each bite. Treat the moment as if you will describe to someone exactly how the food tastes like. By doing this, it helps you keep the focus on the food you eat and appreciate different taste, even the most unpleasant.

Create a mealtime and adhere to it. Avoid eating when you are doing something else; also, this prevents overindulging and helps you measure the quantity as well as eat to satisfaction and not leisure. Multitasking, as you eat, can lead to overeating or indulging in unhealthy foods.

Respond to hunger and satisfaction. When you are hungry eat do not deny your body food, this also applies to when you are full; you should stop eating. Listen and communicate with your body whatever it is telling you to respond appropriately.

Know how different kinds of food make you feel. This is after you eat them. This statement mostly responds to questions like, which meal makes you tired or energized? Avoid food that makes you tired since they reduce the body's metabolism.

Learn to forgive yourself for overindulging even when you are not hungry. The food that you ate because you wanted to but made you tired just forget about them and continue with the food that keeps you energized. Understand that you are not perfect and are bound to be tempted to eat the foods you don't want to eat. When you give in to temptation, forgive yourself, and move on.

Spend time and make responsible food choices, always plan for the kind of foods you'll eat in advance. If you can't do this all the time, make a weekly or daily meal plan.

Acknowledge your food cravings. By doing this, you will be able to resist your craving by understanding that it is reasonable to crave, but you do not have to give in to all types of cravings.

We can design specific techniques and practices concerning mindful eating, meditating, and intuitive eating. By these techniques, we get to have a healthy and productive relationship with regards to food and thereby to eliminate any bad feelings associated with diet and our eating habits. The result of this is healthy weight loss though this should not be the key focus; it should serve more as a reward. If we focus on weight loss as the primary goal, then we may be distracted and not have a focused mind during meditation. When eating, though, you should eat because you are hungry and need to satisfy yourself. Do not eat because you are stressed at work, stressed with family issues, so you need to eat to forget about your stress. Meditation practices help you love your body and be in control of your mind and the decisions you make.

General Health Affirmation

They are statements, phrases, or words that you use in your daily life. Their main task is to give you that maximum motivation in everything that you do. Remember, you always speak these words to yourself. Phrases like this include;

"I can radiate confidence." Confidence refers to the ability to show boldness in what you are doing. You must now be in a position to radiate not only faith but also grace and beauty. Virtues like these are highly significant since they will always guide you daily. You will feel relaxed, motivated, and have the urge to be successful in life. Your health improves, and you will be able to see this in your body image. Elements of grace and beauty will affirm you to your real-life situations. You will be able to maintain this kind of morale, which will eventually help you to make correct decisions on your healthy food. It is good to state that choosing a healthy diet is not only useful to your life but also economical. A proper diet, too, results in an accelerated appetite and urge even to eat more. Healthy food is always good for your body as it supplies you with enough nutrients. Nutrients have the power of smoldering your body, thus improving your body image.

"Every cell within my body accepts good health." You must ascertain yourself always with these words. Good health will always make your whole body vibrates. It is now up to you to concentrate on maintaining good health throughout. You can do this by choosing healthy food from the stores. Healthy eating includes plant-based diets that have less content of meat. The healthy meal plan also incorporates a large intake of water, daily exercises, and eating healthy. All these nourish your body cells, making them carry out their work accordingly. Your motivation to eat every day will develop suddenly, especially when you have all these healthy food at your doorstep. In the long-run period, your body weight reduces due to the assimilation of a healthy diet. Fortunately, in the end, your body image improves, leading to shedding off some pounds.

You must love and show some respect for your body. Your body is built up with so much complexity that when you fail to prove it, love, you can even fail. Show some love to your body by providing everything that it needs.

The body needs nourishment, which comes from food. Choose as healthy as possible food. Healthy food will offer your body that glimmering natural look. You will also reduce weight, thus improving your body image. Elements of love, respect, and other virtues always act as stimuli that help you to achieve much in your body. You will realize that your weight reduces without facing difficulties in the process. Reduction in weight will come as a result of choosing wisely the correct diet and using an affirmation to accelerate their intake in your body. Another general health affirmation is to be in a situation where you can choose issues like health and wellness, and shun or shy off boring workouts, restrictive diets, and so on. I know you might love workouts, but some exercises are just unpleasant. Instead of helping you get over your weight, they will load you with exhaustion, bruises, and other minor injuries. Again, there are restrictive diets that you need to shy off. Eating meat-related meals, completely processed flour, and relying much on junk dishes will only affect you negatively. It is because of this that you choose your body health and its wellness. You can improve your body health by deciding on a healthy diet. Your welfare, too, is paramount. It matters a lot not only to you but also to your general economic status. Making these choices will accelerate your need to have healthy food at your disposal. As a result, your motivation to eat healthy increases a notch higher. All these will lead to improved body image with a decrease in your weight.

Transcendental Meditation and Weight Loss

Meditation is generally utilized as an unwinding instrument, similar to a back rub for the psyche. What's more, much the same as there are numerous approaches to create an organic product serving of mixed greens; meditation accompanies an assortment of systems. One specific sort called Transcendental Meditation (TM) has earned the distinction since the 1960s after a celebrated musical crew called "The Beatles" began rehearsing it.

Here are the means to rehearse TM:

- Take a seat, assuming a comfortable position. Do not cross your arms or legs.

- Make sure your eyes are closed. Take several deep breaths to bring the body into relaxation.

- Open your eyes shut them once more. Your eyes will assume this state for the whole 20-minute duration.

- Decide on the mantra to recite in your mind.

- When you notice that the mind has started to wander, refocus your attention back to the mantra.

- After the whole duration is over, slowly move your toes and fingers to return you to reality.

- Open your eyes.

- If you do not feel prepared to go on with your day, sit for a longer duration.

- Indeed, you might think about how TM will help with weight decrease. As per research directed on veterans experiencing PTSD, when the psyche rises above, the body comes into an expression far more profound than even profound rest and goes there undeniably more rapidly. Stress prompts a characteristic instrument, which is intended for our assurance to endure.

This pressure logically triggers various exercises to counter the response:

- The front piece of the cerebrum will be detached, the part which is liable for drive control.

- The creation of the bliss hormone "dopamine" diminishes (the pressure hormone "cortisol" increments.

- Individuals under pressure are less and less able to tune in to the reasonable needs of the body.

Rising above is fundamentally the contrary experience of pressure, and that way, it will have the opposite impacts. The subsequent harmony enables the body likewise to increase exceptionally profound rest (further than rest), in which it can disintegrate even its most profound anxieties aggregated because of life's most exceedingly terrible injuries. As we develop revived and renewed from the quietness of meditation, this can deliver different emotional upgrades in any part of our life.

Mindful Eating

We eat mindlessly. The principal explanation behind our awkwardness with nourishment and eating is that we have overlooked how to be available. Careful eating is the act of developing a receptive familiarity with how the food we eat influences one's body, sentiments, brain, and all around us. The training improves our comprehension of what to eat, how to eat, the amount to eat, and why we eat what we eat. When eating carefully, we are entirely present and relish each chomp - connecting every one of our faculties to value the nourishment. Past simple tastes, we see the appearance, sounds, scents, and surfaces of our food, just as our mind's reaction to these perceptions.

Steps to Mindful Eating

Watch Your Shopping List

Shopping mindfully, – purchasing sound nourishments that are reasonably delivered and bundled – is a significant piece of the training.

One thing you will probably find about careful eating is that entire nourishments are more dynamic and heavenly than you may have given them acknowledgment for.

Learn How to Eat Slower

Eating gradually does not need to mean taking it to limits. It is a smart thought to remind yourself, and your family, that eating is not a race.

Setting aside the effort to relish and make the most of your nourishment is perhaps the most advantageous thing you can do. You are bound to see when you are full, you'll bite your food more and consequently digest it all the more effectively, and you'll likely end up seeing flavors you may find some way, or another have missed.

Eat When Necessary

However, it might take some training to locate that sweet spot between being eager and hungry to the point that you need to breathe in a dinner.

Additionally, tune in to your body and get familiar with the distinction between being physically eager and sincerely ravenous. On the off chance that you skip dinners, you might be so anxious to get anything in your stomach that your first need fills the void instead of making the most of your nourishment.

Enjoy Your Senses

The vast majority partner eating with simple taste and many eat so carelessly that even the taste buds get quick work. Be that as it may, eating is a blessing to a higher number of faculties than simply taste. When you are cooking, serving, and eating your nourishment, be mindful of shading, surface, fragrance, and even the sounds various nourishments make as you set them up. As you bite your food, take a stab at distinguishing every one of the fixings, particularly seasonings. Eat with your fingers to give your feeling of touch some good times. By drawing in various faculties, the entire experience turns out to be significantly more completely fulfilling.

Keep off Distractions

Our day by day lives are brimming with interruptions, and it is normal for families to eat with the TV boom or one relative or another tinkering with their iPhone. Think about making family supper time, which should be eaten together, a hardware-free zone. This does not mean eating alone peacefully; careful eating can be a tremendous mutual encounter. It just means you do not eat before the TV, while driving, on the PC, on your telephone, and so on. Eating before the TV is the national hobby, however, simply consider how effectively it empowers mindless eating.

Stop when you are full

The issue with astounding nourishment is that it tends to be challenging to quit eating by its very nature. Eating gradually will enable you to feel full before overeating. Still, on the other hand, it is imperative to be mindful of segment size and tune in to your body for when it starts disclosing to you it has had enough. Gorging may feel great at the time; however, it is awkward for a short time and is commonly not beneficial for the body.

Meditating to Heal Your Relationship With Food

The capacity to hold a full scope of various feelings for the day is a test for a considerable lot of us. We simply need to feel upbeat, yet the test is to locate that mystical parity of all that we experience, decipher, and do. The most natural history of past weight reduction endeavors is ceaseless confinements, which requires self-discipline and force. This perspective has a negative turn and does not draw out the best of us.

Mindful Eating Meditation Script

Start by interfacing with your breath and body, feel your feet on the ground, and notice your involvement at this time. With your mindfulness at this time, see any contemplations, sensations, or, then again, feelings you are encountering.

Tune into the mindfulness or impression that you have in your collection of inclination eager, parched, or perhaps feeling full. On the off chance that you would eat or drink something at present, what is your body hungry for? What is it eager for? Simply focus and notice with mindfulness the vibes that give you this data. (Interruption)

Presently, get your regard for the thing in your hand and envision that you see it just because. See with interest as you focus and notice the shading, shape, surface, and size. Is there something else that you notice, sense, or feel? (Interruption)

You are allowed to alter the procedure just as you would prefer.

Utilizing a care-eating exercise is just a single piece of a caring way to deal with your eating regimen. The freeing intensity of care produces further results when you start to give careful consideration to your contemplations, feelings, and real sensations, all of which lead us to eat. Attention (mindfulness) is the establishment that numerous individuals have been missing for defeating nourishment longings, addictive eating, voraciously consuming food, enthusiastic eating, and stress eating.

Foods to Eat for Deeper Meditation

Meditation can be extreme. Take out every single stray idea? Concentrate just on your breath? Sit still for (at least) 10 minutes one after another? In any case, we are increasingly finding out that rehearsing everyday meditation has such a large number of astonishing advantages, from helping us become progressively empathetic to empowering us to be increasingly quiet, adoring, happy, excusing, and liberal.

Green Tea

Numerous old societies related to Tea with long life and wellbeing. Starting in China, it has been utilized as medication for a great many years. Green Tea has not exclusively been filling our mugs for quite a while yet has played a job as a fundamental fixing in numerous a sweet.

It has been the subject in various therapeutic and logical investigations to decide if it is since quite a while ago, toted medical advantages convey any legitimacy.

Tomatoes

A lot of vitamin C, which is generally viewed as valuable in bringing down your pressure. As per an investigation led in Japan, members who ate tomatoes over six times each week had an essentially lower danger of framing discouragement.

Specialists are attempting to make sense of whether lycopene, the synthetic segment that makes tomatoes dark red, legitimately influences psychological prosperity.

Lemon or Lemon Water

Lemons are generally plentiful in nutrients and minerals, especially nutrient C, a cell reinforcement that lifts the resistant framework, ensures against cardiovascular sickness, and helps avert malignant growth. Lemons likewise animate vitality and can help upgrade your state of mind. How? The two lemons and limes are one of only a handful couple of nourishments that contain more negative charged particles than positive ones, which gives your body an increase in vitality when it enters your stomach-related tract.

Nuts

Brimming with cell reinforcement Vitamin E and zinc, nuts, such as almonds, pistachios, and pecans, are useful for boosting the insusceptible framework. They likewise contain a lot of B-Vitamins, which help you oversee pressure and sadness. Scientists have demonstrated that nuts improve our cerebrums' capacity to tackle issues, one more significant piece of meditation.

Vegetables and Whole Fruits

Eating an eating regimen wealthy in whole foods grown from the ground is probably the best thing you can accomplish for your body. The equivalent is similarly valid for the brain. Root vegetables, including sweet potatoes, squash, and carrots, are pressed with a wide range of nutrients and minerals.

CHAPTER 12:

How to Practice Every Day

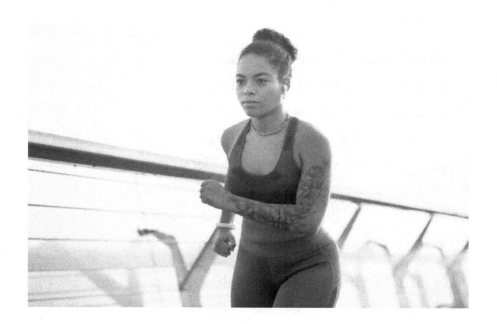

What is the secret to getting rid of weight problems? I am going to tell you. The trick is breaking the old subconscious blocks, generating new patterns of thought and harmonizing the conscious and subconscious mind. Hypnosis will help you conquer the subconscious bloc obstacles.

You'll feel better. They're going to feel in control. You'll feel sure to be able to control your weight with encouragement and determination to keep up with your weight loss goals. Hypnosis has none of the negative or harmful side effects of diet pills or surgery. If you choose a successful diet and exercise plan and then reprogram your mind to make it no longer challenging but simple, pleasant and efficient to follow your food and fitness programmer, you will certainly succeed.

Have fun exercising and eating healthy, so you can stop causing self-induced tension, stress and discouragement. You will start doing the things that will help you in your aim of being safe and losing weight, obviously. You need to get rid of the unhealthy habits of thought that make you overweight. These thought patterns, which are stored in your subconscious mind, must be replaced with healthier thoughts and healthy behaviors so that you can instinctively do what you are expected to do without ever thinking twice about it.

Does that sound tricky? In reality it's much less complicated than you would imagine. All you need is 10 to 20 minutes a day for a total of 21 days (the amount of time it takes to build a habit).

You can now have what it takes to speedily program your mind to lose weight. You see, hypnosis is one of today's world's most overlooked and powerful methods for self-change.

When you say "hypnosis," most people think of magic shows in Vegas or stupid acts on stage. Those on stage were chosen especially because of their susceptibility to suggestion. They wouldn't do anything that they normally wouldn't do on stage. For the publicity they receive, they really "do not mind" behaving stupidly on stage. If they don't perform, they know they're going to be taken off the stage and back to the seat. There could not be anything further from the facts. In theory, hypnosis is a very comfortable state of mind in which you become more receptive to suggestions. During the day, you usually go through hypnosis many times.

If the use of hypnosis for treating illness has been accepted by major medical societies, imagine how amazingly successful and beneficial it is when coping with thought patterns that stand in the way of the healthy body you deserve. The use of hypnosis has been used for more than half a century to treat illness. In addition, in 1955 the British Medical Association approved the hypnotherapy use. Its use was approved in 1958 by the American Medical Association.

In a 9-week trial-weight management group study (one using hypnosis and one not using it), the hypnosis group has continued to get results in the two-year follow-up, while the non-hypnosis group did not show any further results (Journal of Clinical Psychology, 1985). The groups using hypnosis lost an average of 16 pounds in a sample of 60 participants, while the other group lost an average of just 0.5 pounds (Journal of Consulting & Clinical Psychology, 1986). Multiple studies showed that the addition of hypnosis increased the weight loss by an average of 97% during treatment and, more importantly, the efficacy increased by more than 146% after treatment. Hypnosis is known to perform much better over time (Journal of Consulting & Clinical Psychology, 1996). "The best way to break bad habits is by hypnosis," even Newsweek Magazine said.

Whether you want to use audio tapes or CD's for hypnosis, review the script used to determine if the suggestions make sense to you. Make sure there are no suggestions that are negative.

The subconscious will not hear "no" or "no" so the suggestion 's emphasis would be: I do not consume fattening foods. This will give you your objective in the opposite direction. Just use constructive feedback. "I just eat fresh foods that make me feel solid, safe and happy" is much better.

When you get up in the morning and before going to bed in the evening is the best time for your mind to accept these positive suggestions. You need a quiet room where nothing won't bother you. When you're getting a lot of action in your house, you may need to find a room where you can shut the door and get undisturbed. It only lasts for 10 to 20 minutes.

Hypnosis is not a one-time fix for most people. The Hypnosis results are cumulative. The more post-hypnotic suggestions are applied to the hypnosis, the more permanent the results become. So, few people are likely to get hypnotized once to avoid smoking or lose weight. We usually create a new habit if they do, to replace the one they just quit. Most people who quit smoking begin overeating. We were replacing only one undesirable habit with another. Unless the root(s) of the problem is found there would be no need to add another habit.

Having a specialist skilled in hypnosis and weight loss struggles could prove useful. Working with a specialist will help you understand the earlier programming and remove it.

Especially with weight loss, use relaxation and self-hypnosis every morning and evening to be effective, changing and perfecting your suggestions while you lose weight. Upon reaching the weight you are comfortable with; you might want to add other goals along with strengthening your healthy eating and exercising habits.

You will need to start with the full relaxation at first, but after a week or so you will be able to go very quickly into the altered relaxed state by counting down from 10 to 1. Always end your session with a suggestion that makes you feel good, better than ever, relaxed and either alert, clear-headed, refreshed and full of morning energy or relaxed and able to sleep soundly when you go to bed at night.

Keep a pen and paper close by to write down any insights that come to mind while listening to your suggestions or reading them. You can recall things that you were told as a child that now influence your behavior.

CHAPTER 13:

Love your Body

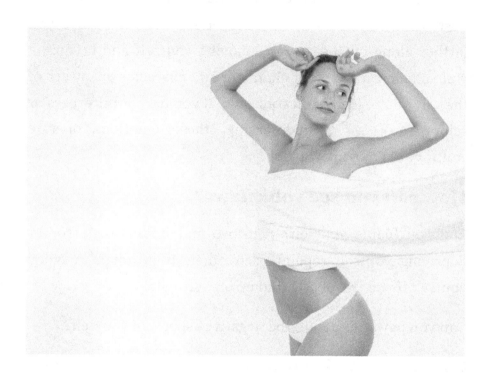

The majority of individuals don't think very much about self-improvement. We'd love to assist you to indulge in such a notion and find out just how much you can enjoy yourself. It's a requirement for accepting and creating your ideal weight and everything else that's fantastic for you. Just being conscious of the idea of self-help can move you farther along on the way of enjoying yourself and accepting yourself as you are. Your character and character are aware of the way you're feeling on your own. If you harbor bitterness or remorse, or sense undeserving, these emotions operate contrary to enjoying yourself.

How can you see your flaws?

Can you blame yourself? Self-love and finding an error or depriving yourself repaint each other. It is tough to enjoy yourself if you frequently find errors ultimately.

Can you pay attention to the negative aspects of yourself?

Can you end up making self-deprecating statements, such as "I am not intelligent enough to..." or even "I am not great enough to..."?

Can you punish yourself or refuse yourself?

Can you establish boundaries with individuals who represent your very own moral and ethical criteria and your values and beliefs?

Look at the mirror. How do you feel about yourself? Can you smile or frown?

Which are you about the continuum of self?

Are you currently respectful and admiring?

Are you critical and judgmental, or would you love yourself for who you are?

Have you been caring and caring for this individual who you see?

If you're ambivalent, then contemplate these concerns further. Be truthful with yourself. Have a conversation on your own. Take a sincere look at yourself. Do not just examine your own body; examine your wisdom, your soul, your own emotions, along with your own heart. Know that: By enjoying yourself, you love yourself. If there's something that you can't accept on your own, be aware you could change that idea, and alter it to make anything you want, such as your ideal weight.

The power of self-love and forgiveness

Have a Look at These characteristics? Are these familiar to you? It is the way it will feel for those who like yourself:

You genuinely feel happy and accepting your world, even though you might not agree with everything within it.

You're compassionate with your flaws or less-than-perfect behaviors, understanding that you're capable of improving and changing.

You mercifully love compliments and feel joyful inside.

You frankly see your flaws and softly accept them learn to alter them.

You accept all of the goodness that comes your way.

You honor the great qualities and the fantastic qualities of everybody around you.

You look at the mirror and smile

Many confound self-love with becoming arrogant and greedy. But some individuals are so caught up in themselves they make the tag of being egotistical and thinking just of these. We do not find that as a healthful indulgence, however, as a character that's not well balanced in enjoying love and loving others. It's not selfish to get things your way; however, it's egotistical to insist that everybody else can see them your way too. The Dalai Lama states, "If you do not enjoy yourself, then you can't love other people. You won't have the capacity to appreciate others. If you don't have any empathy on your own, then you aren't capable of developing empathy for others." Dr. Karl Menninger, a psychologist, states it this way: "Self-love isn't opposed to this love of different men and women. You cannot truly enjoy yourself and get yourself a favor with no people a favor, and vice versa." We're referring to the healthiest type of self-indulgence that simplifies the solution to accepting your best good.

Have a better look at the way you see your flaws and blame yourself. Self-love and finding an error or depriving yourself aren't in any way compatible. If you suppress or refuse to enjoy yourself, you're in danger of paying too much focus on your flaws that are a sort of self-loathing. You Don't Want to place focus on negative aspects of yourself, for holding these ideas in your mind, and You're giving them the psychological energy which brings that result or leaves it actual.

Self-hypnosis can help you use your mind-body to make new and much more loving ideas and beliefs on your own. It helps your mind-body create and take fluctuations in the patterns of feeling and thinking about what has been for you for quite a while, and which aren't helpful for you. The trancework about the sound incorporates many positive suggestions to change your ideas, emotions, and beliefs in alignment with your ideal weight.

Forgiving Yourself for Your Dietary Mistakes

Forgiveness is an underrated and essential element of weight loss. Often, people that are within the position of wanting or wanting to reduce and fail to acknowledge the very fact that they need been feeling incredibly frustrated with themselves. Anger, frustration, disappointment, and sadness directed at yourself once you are on this journey are all incredibly normal feelings to possess.

They can even be painful and overwhelming if you are doing not take the time to acknowledge them, forgive yourself, and heal them as you experience them.

You may end up feeling angry, frustrated, disappointed, or sad that you simply let yourself gain such a lot of weight. You'll fail to acknowledge the very fact that it had been not intentional, or that it had causes that were beyond your control, mainly if your weight gain was associated with medical conditions or a scarcity of education around healthy eating.

Regardless of what causes you to gain weight, you'll feel contempt for yourself for "allowing" it to happen, which may make it difficult for you to plan to lose weight.

When you sit in anger and frustration with yourself, it is often difficult to simply accept yourself as you're now and work toward improving your wellbeing through weight loss. Forgiving yourself for not knowing better or for not doing better, or maybe forgiving yourself for blaming yourself for something that was beyond your control, is vital.

The more you'll forgive yourself, the more likely you're to acknowledge that your weight is some things you would like to figure on. Through that, you'll be ready to work on weight loss from a peaceful frame of mind.

Studies have shown that those that accept themselves as they're and forgive their mistakes are more likely to lose the surplus weight and keep it off than those that refuse to forgive themselves. Refusing to forgive yourself can create a huge amount of stress inside you that creates it difficult for you to remain focused on exercising, eating healthy, and improving your wellness. Many of us find that this difficulty in forgiving ourselves worsens their self-esteem and self-confidence, which keeps them within the unhealthy cycle of behaviors and patterns that cause their weight gain in the first place. If you would like to beat these cycles, you would like to be willing to forgive yourself for your past choices, mistakes, and experiences which will or might not are beyond your control.

Another area where you would like to master forgiveness is within the process of change. As you progress faraway from old habits and behaviors and into a replacement way of taking care of your body, you're bound to make mistakes.

You are getting to have days or maybe weeks where you fall back to old patterns.

Some people even fall back to old patterns and stay trapped in them for years. This fact happens because they're unwilling to forgive themselves for creating an error, then they fall back to the cycle of contempt and low self-esteem and self-worth.

If you would like to be ready to continue moving forward together with your wellness and to leap back on target as quickly as possible, you would like to be willing to forgive yourself for any mistakes you create. This way means anytime you overeat, engage in an old eating pattern, choose an unhealthy food choice, or otherwise make a "mistake" in your diet, and you forgive yourself. Upon forgiving yourself, confirm that you also plan to take that have under consideration so that you'll make better choices. Make an honest effort to try to do better next time so that whenever you forgive yourself, you give yourself a reason to believe that your commitment to yourself genuinely means something. When you can forgive yourself and believe that your commitment to bettering yourself and your life means something, you start to create your self-esteem. Through that, things like portion control begin to become easier, and you discover yourself naturally gravitating toward taking better care of yourself.

How Does It Feel to Love Yourself?

Have a look at These features. Are these familiar to you? It is the way it should feel if you like yourself:

You genuinely feel happy and accepting your world, even though you might not agree with everything within it.

You're compassionate with your flaws or less-than-perfect behaviors, understanding that you're capable of improving and changing.

You mercifully love compliments and feel joyful inside.

You frankly see your flaws and softly accept them learn to alter them.

You accept all of the goodness that comes your way.

You honor the great qualities and the fantastic qualities of everybody around you.

You look at the mirror and smile (at least all the period).

Many confuse self-love with becoming arrogant and greedy. But some individuals are so caught up in themselves, they make the tag of being egotistical and thinking just of these. We do not find that as a healthful self-indulgent, however, as a character which isn't well balanced in enjoying itself love and loving others.

It isn't selfish to get things your way; however, it's egotistical to insist that everybody else can see them your way too. The Dalai Lama states, "If you do not enjoy yourself, then you can't love other people. You won't have the capacity to appreciate others. If you don't have any empathy on your own, then you aren't capable of developing empathy for others" Dr. Karl Menninger, a psychologist, states it this way: "Self-love isn't opposed to this love of different men and women. You can't truly enjoy yourself and get yourself a favor with no people a favor, and vice versa." We're referring to the healthiest type of self-indulgence that simplifies the solution to accepting your best good.

Just take a better look at the way you see your flaws and blame yourself. Self-love and finding an error or depriving yourself aren't in any way compatible. If you deny enjoying yourself, you're in danger of paying too much focus on your flaws that are a sort of self-loathing. You don't wish to place focus on negative aspects of yourself, for by keeping these ideas in your mind, you're giving them the psychological energy which brings that result or leaves it actual.

Self-love is positive energy. Blame, criticism, and faultfinding are energy. Self-hypnosis can help you utilize your mind-body to make new and much more loving ideas and beliefs on your own. It helps your mind-body create and take fluctuations in the patterns of feeling and thinking which have been for you for quite a while, and which aren't helpful for you. The trancework about the sound incorporates many positive suggestions to shift your ideas, emotions, and beliefs in alignment together with your ideal weight.

A Vital goal for all these positive hypnotic suggestions is the innermost feeling of enjoying yourself. If your self-loving feelings are constant with your ideal weight, then it is going to occur with increased ease. But if you harbor bitterness or remorse, or sense undeserving, these emotions operate contrary to enjoying yourself enough to think and take your ideal weight. Lucille Ball stated it well: "Love yourself first and everything falls in line" The hypnotic suggestions about the sound are directions for change led to the maximum "internal" degree of mind-body or unconscious. However, the "outer" changes in life action should also happen.

Many weight reduction methods you have been using might appear to be a lot of work. We suggest that by adopting a mindset that's without the psychological pressure related to "needing to," "bad or good," or even "simple or difficult," with no judgment in any way, the fluctuations could be joyous.

Yes, even joyous. It produces the whole journey of earning adjustments and shifting easier. The term "a labor of love" implies you enjoy doing this so much it isn't labor or responsibility. The "labor" of organizing a family feast in a vacation season, volunteering at a hospital or school, or even buying a gift for someone very particular can appear effortless. Here is the mindset that will assist you in following some weight loss methods. We invite you to place yourself in the situation of getting adored.

You're doing so to you. Loving yourself eliminates the job, and that means it is possible to relish your advancement toward a lifestyle that encourages your ideal weight. Think about some action that you like to perform. Imagine yourself performing this action today. Notice that whenever you're doing something which you love to perform, you're feeling energized and beautiful, and some other attempt comes out by enjoyment. What is going on at these times is you see it absolutely "loving what you're doing." Sometimes, we recommend that you also find that as "enjoying yourself doing this." Maybe by directing a more favorable attitude toward enjoying yourself, you'll end up enjoying what you're doing.

Conclusion

There are many reasons why someone should use hypnosis to lose weight. First, hypnosis is often successful when all other avenues of weight, health, and fitness have failed, and that's for a good reason!

The problem is not the method or even the plan you are using to achieve it. The problem is in your mind. If you want to lose real body fat, reduce weight, make your ideal shape, and maintain your new look, it is essential to change your attitude towards food and exercise, and your behavior towards both.

The best hypnosis programs for weight loss may require you to understand and replicate those mental processes used by people who have lost weight already. It might be tough leaving your comfort zone, but hypnosis will help you to reprogram your mind and install new thoughts that will become automatic habits once you identify the right behavior perfect for achieving your goal.

Eating less and adequately, or exercise following a schedule won't be a dream anymore: hypnosis enhances and strengthens your will.

So, if you are worried about being overweight now, there is nothing wrong with undergoing hypnosis. After all, you have nothing to lose

Ultimately, hypnosis, both in a professional or home setting, has the potential to help with weight loss. According to Vanderbilt University, hypnosis works best for individuals who need to lose low-to-moderate amounts of weight.

It doesn't mean that you shouldn't attempt it but talk with your doctor about working it into a routine that incorporates other weight loss behaviors. It requires a various number of hypnosis sessions by a hypnotherapist. It may take a long time before professional therapy alters your attitudes and actions, and it may take a while before changed behaviors become a habit.

Try not to get discouraged with little change. If nothing else, regular hypnosis sessions may help ease pressure and help you learn to relax, reducing your need to eat in emotional situations. Because hypnosis is probably not going to deal with the issue all by itself, consider keeping a food and exercise journal.

Also, record how long you practiced and what kind of activity you did. This log considers you accountable for poor decisions and allows you to distinguish patterns in your eating and exercise habits that may counteract healthy weight loss. When you identify these patterns, you'll have a venturing off point for your next hypnosis session, as far as critical thinking and behavior modifications may assist you with weight loss.

Regardless of how you approach hypnosis, its advantage may be what you have to finally lose that abundance of weight and carry on with a healthier life—good karma helps with using hypnosis to achieve your weight loss goals. Add up many small strides for weight loss success.

The more you practice the meditations we've given to you, the easier it will be to discover the success you've been waiting for. After a complicated diet, again and again, getting nowhere is an ideal opportunity to accept what isn't right about our mindset.

A perfect way to turn your mood around is to rework it through meditation. Tune in to these at whatever point you're home and find the opportunity. If you're exhausted, why not take a few minutes to relax and pull yourself together?

Whatever strategy for eating healthy you may pick; these meditations and trances will help you stop gorging and think it is easier to eat healthily and practice naturally. Recollect that it takes over one attempt and that you should practice it regularly, not once a month. When you can incorporate these snapshots of relaxation into your routine, it will help them work better.

All the best

EXTREME WEIGHT LOSS HYPNOSIS FOR WOMEN

HOW TO BURN FAT AND LOSE WEIGHT QUICKLY USING GASTRIC BAND HYPNOSIS AND GUIDED MEDITATION TECHNIQUES.

Eva Ruell

Introduction

Have you at any point heard how Hypnosis has helped other people reach their goals?

Maybe you have even thought about various ways you might use self-hypnosis to make changes in your own life for the better but have failed to get enough resources to do so.

The world relies on scientific evidence for almost everything. From car brakes to food hygiene, practically all safety mechanisms, from gas appliance maintenance to front door locks – rely on scientific evidence. Given that you follow the generally accepted scientific advice, you don't tend to rely on anyone's gut feeling or anecdotal evidence when it comes to the essential aspects of everyday life.

In a supersized world, people have too many options to eat and drink, but what is behind overweight is often more than the desire for a wide variety of potato chips. The diet has developed around obesity, forcing overweight people to pay a high price for expensive and risky diets, pills, or operations. Many have to cut out carbs or fats, take medications or injections, perform surgeries, or drink miracle potions. Many dieters lose weight temporarily but don't change the mindset that contributes to weight gain. The result is that after all the hard work and potentially spending thousands of dollars, most dieters regain their weight and feel even more frustrated.

The healthiest and most effective way to lose weight is not the fastest. For those who want to maintain a healthy weight and healthily lose body fat, weight loss hypnosis is what you should consider.

Weight loss should be smooth without constant hunger and constant food cravings. Weight loss hypnosis is an effective way to lose weight because it is easy to retrain your subconscious, and you can see the results immediately. Weight loss hypnosis can help you change your emotions and control your low diet.

Like all Hypnosis, weight loss hypnosis proposes weight loss while people are relaxed, as long as the suggestions correspond to what the person wants to do. Part of the focus is on changing preferences and choices for a better alimentation and to overcome appetite.

Since many dieters have negative thinking patterns that encourage them to use junk food to change their feelings, Hypnosis for weight loss also helps you see yourself as a healthy person who does not need food to change anything. You learn to see changes in eating habits not as a hardship but as empowerment because that is what you want to do in the first place.

You are getting tired. While the vast majority have the picture of the turning high contrast wheel when they consider subliminal therapy, this isn't an exact depiction. Hypnosis has been mainstream both dramatically and remedially for quite a long time and has taken on numerous structures. All the more, as of late, Hypnosis has gained decent notoriety in clinical practices for a horde of reasons. This is what you have to think about the training and why you ought to get mesmerized.

Hypnosis is a cycle of conscious mindfulness where mental portrayals supersede physiology, recognition, and conduct, referred to by numerous reliable clinical diaries. It isn't some sort of magic, and it doesn't transform you into a robot. However, it's critical to take note that entranced individuals are not dozing or oblivious. Instead, it's a hyper-mindful and hyper-responsive mental state where the brain is profoundly open to recommendations. Subsequently, an individual under Hypnosis has full concentration without doubt or ecological mindfulness.

This book contains proven steps and strategies for reprogramming your subconscious mind using self-hypnosis and unleashing the hidden power within which you have been longing.

CHAPTER 14:

What is Hypnosis for Weight Loss?

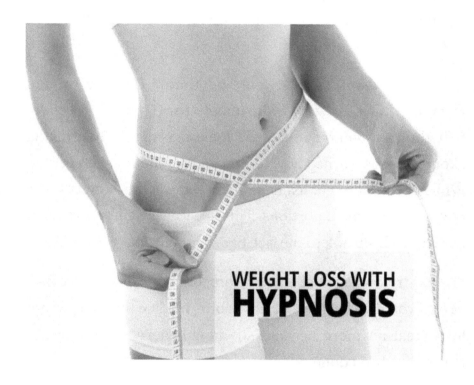

It's using hypnosis techniques to allow you to lose weight. It's a way to shed a few extra pounds. But most of the time, it is paired with a diet plan. It would help if you continued an excellent regimen of food, followed by moderate exercise. But this will allow you to lose weight faster, and if you're a person who has cravings for things, this will help you immensely.

A perfect example of this would-be Marion Corns, a woman from the United Kingdom who underwent Hypnosis to believe that she has undergone Gastric Bypass Surgery. By thinking about this, she learned how to control the amount she's eating. While she used to eat as many food plates as she wanted, she now only eats small portions. This is because she believes that her stomach shrunk to the size of a golf ball!

She has tried many diet plans before, but none of them worked as she would go back to her old habits, but she tells herself not to overeat anymore because she now believes that a gastric bypass has been done.

What's impressive, too, is the fact that she didn't undergo gastric bypass, and yet, she's able to reap the benefits. An operation would have cost her a little more than $7,000. She didn't shelve out that cash, but now, she has lost a lot of pounds—and that's all because of Hypnosis!

She underwent five sessions of gastric Hypnosis in a hospital in Spain. She was already supposed to go through the operation there, but then she found out that that the clinic also gives Gastric Hypnosis sessions, so she decided to go for that one. After five sessions, she felt like her stomach was tightening, and every time she tries to eat more than she should, she feels like she's going to throw up.

According to her, what happened was that she went through Cognitive Behavioral Therapy, which could also be a form of Hypnosis. Now, she feels like she finally fits in with society, and she no longer feels like she has to hide from people.

So how exactly does it work?

It's best to do this when you have a window of time ready for you to take care of this issue. You'll want at least thirty minutes of quiet time to handle these cravings, ideally an hour at most. You will be running some pretty heavy matters, so making sure that you're relaxed and able to return to reality before and after the Hypnosis will make it all the better.

Hypnosis works in a way that can help someone naturally feel that he is making the right choice when it comes to food. Does this mean taking away someone's willpower? It doesn't. It merely means helping someone feel better about using his will as far as food choices are concerned.

After all, losing weight is not about getting rid of something we do not want or need. People have become so focused on exercise routines and obsessed with 'healthy' foods. Of course, it is perfectly alright to pay attention to these things, but it is also important to train our brains. That is where Hypnosis comes in. Hypnosis can help in such a way that a person can create a new relationship with his body and food. Rather than taking away someone's willpower, Hypnosis can be used successfully to reinforce someone's power to choose and be more honest with these choices. For instance, you know you can always have chocolate cake, and you can have as much as you want, but do you have to have it? You know you want it, but do you need it?

There are various approaches to using Hypnosis for weight loss. Do not focus on one aspect. Choose a set of approaches relevant to that person.

Use suggestions to help the person envision the body he wants and the level of health and fitness he wants to achieve.

Use positive suggestions to help someone maximize his motivation to eat healthily.

Encourage the person to level up his fat-burning metabolism. Provide specific cues that will remind him to exercise. For instance, you can suggest that his legs will feel restless at a particular time each day, which means it is time to exercise.

Metaphors can also be used successfully. For example, you can conjure up an image in the person's mind of a sculptor facing a shapeless rock. In order to uncover the real form of that rock, the sculptor must work on it little by little, carefully and patiently. When the real form is revealed, he can get rid of the excess and needless rocks.

Another imagery you can use to help someone lose weight is to guide him into visualizing that he is wearing a fat suit. Guide him into imagining that he is able to discard layers from his fat suit. Reinforce that feeling of relief as he removes one layer at a time until the suit is in the 'right' size, the way he wants his body to look. Help the person focus not just on numbers and weight but also on health and fitness.

Help the person make a distinction between real food and fake food, the ones that are good for him and the ones that aren't.

Use a hypnotic journey metaphor. Suggest that in each step of the journey, he feels lighter and better about himself. Allow him to think about what he's wearing as he gets farther in the journey.

Use disassociation to help this person see himself in the future when he eats well, exercises regularly, looking slimmer and feeling much lighter.

Use age progression. Take him into the future where he has become slimmer. Suggest that he goes back in time from the future and remembers exactly what he needed to do to make this happen and how easy and effortless it was.

Help the person realize that when he exercises more, his will to exercise becomes greater and it becomes much easier.

Help him remember that when he feels the desire to eat unhealthily or consume food when he is not hungry, he is not reaching his goal. Let him imagine how it will make him feel to not reach his goal.

Does it Work?

The effectiveness varies from person to person. It will help you, and, on average, a person loses about six pounds. You might lose more, but you might not lose as much as expected. If you're trying to lose a ton of weight, this might not help. But, if you're looking to help eliminate cravings in your life and live a healthier lifestyle, then this is definitely the right tool for you. It's a way to help you supplement your exercising plans, and with this, you'll be able to have an even better time when it comes to shedding those pounds fast.

The Benefits

There are other benefits of using Hypnosis for weight loss. The obvious big one is that you lose weight. That's the one people will notice. You'll start to shed those pounds, and you might lose more than you expected. It won't be significant, such as like fifty pounds or more, but if you want to help your body and allow yourself the benefits of being able to control the cravings to lose weight, then this is perfect for you.

Then there are the lasting benefits of it. These are the benefits that you'll get because of the Hypnosis. When you're doing this, you'll be able to tackle those parts of your subconscious that think it's okay to eat when you're stressed, or it'll tell you to eat more than necessary. Sometimes, your mind can be your own worst enemy, and this is certainly one of those times. With Hypnosis for weight loss, you'll allow yourself to handle your body in a positive manner. If you do this, you'll actually allow yourself to control your cravings and desires through the use of Hypnosis. It might seem crazy, but it is possible.

Hypnosis for Weight Loss - What Can Hypnosis Do?

Hypnosis may be defined as a routine inducing an alternate state of awareness, which helps persons become highly sensitive to a hypnotist's suggestions.

This routine has been accepted in psychoanalysis for treating psychic illnesses by revisiting the harmful events which caused them in the past and then by transmitting suggestions created to assist them.

Hypnosis may be used to overcome phobias. Hypnosis may be used to lessen stress or tension. Hypnosis may help you remain calm before a big test and during your big speech. You will most certainly benefit from Hypnosis.

Hypnosis may regulate blood flow and different autonomic functions that are not generally subject to conscious manipulation. The relaxing reaction that occurs with Hypnosis also alters the Neuro-hormonal systems that regulate many body functions.

Hypnosis for weight loss may assist you in passing when everything else has failed. Using Hypnosis, we may aid you to achieve the weight loss that you want. Hypnosis may go straight to the middle of the matter and specialize in replacing particular behavior or habits with healthy choices.

Hypnosis may also be used to transform those who are hurt by anxiety attacks. These are characterized by the inability to concentrate, problems in making decisions, extreme sensitivity, disharmony, sleep interruptions, excessive sweating, and consistent muscle tension.

Hypnosis may aid by giving you coping systems so that you can face them in more appropriate ways whenever stress-inducing situations happen. Hypnosis may be used in many various ways.

Hypnosis may also be a method of pain control, often used with burn victims and women in labor. Hypnosis cannot depose an exercise outline but may implement and strengthen it.

Hypnotic affirmations have a cumulative therapeutic effect in the subconscious part of the mind, with the capability of improving healthy self-esteem. Hypnosis can't make a person to do anything against their will or that contradicts their values.

A Hypnotherapist has ethics that are required to create only those changes that abide by agreed-upon change work.

Hypnosis can help you obtain personal achievements and help you remain motivated toward obtaining those goals. After a few sessions of "hypnosis therapy," you may find more willingness to live and have more energy than ever imagined.

Does Weight Loss Hypnosis Work?

Mesmerizing can be thought of as an ability - a device that individuals use to unwind, change their points of view and sentiments in a more advantageous, progressively positive, and helpful way. All Hypnosis is "self-spellbinding" so the individual is 100% responsible for how it functions and the outcomes. The subliminal specialist resembles a mentor who educates and directs the individual in a loose and simple method of realizing what they need to succeed. This is totally founded on the decision to get in shape the individual makes; in any case, Hypnosis is never a substitute for an individual choice. Neither the subliminal specialist nor Hypnosis itself can "make" an individual do anything. The individual needs to get more fit.

Hypnosis is growing in popularity as a way of treating many different conditions, such as stress, smoking cessation, emotional issues, low self-esteem, fear of public speaking, and the list goes on. One of the most successful uses of Hypnosis is for weight loss. In this article, we will explore why it is gaining popularity and the reasons you should consider it for your weight control goals.

There are three specific reasons you should choose weight loss hypnosis over other weight loss programs.

Any get-healthy plan, paying little heed to what it is, expects you to be fruitful in the brain first before you can bring that accomplishment into physical reality. A decent trance specialist will educate and empower you with self-entrancing so you can generally consider yourself to be effective and stay in a positive mood concerning your weight control.

The brain looks like a muscle, and it takes exercise to get more grounded to ensure control and consistency.

Hypnosis is inexpensive in comparison to all other methods. Consider the price for gastric bypass surgery, for instance, or even special foods or diet drugs your doctor may prescribe.

The prices for some of the various weight loss programs make the fees of a hypnotist seem like nickels in comparison. Plus, you are still going to have to deal with the mind and the motivation factor. Motivation comes and goes in waves like emotions or feelings. We feel super motivated to accomplish all our goals, eat nutritious foods, work out, and improve ourselves. Then there are times you can hit an emotional wall where you feel unmotivated and dive for the first piece of chocolate or apple pie that crosses your path.

With Hypnosis, you can utilize these inner tools to develop the consistent discipline that will not only assist you to lose weight permanently but also help you take those same gifts and apply them to all other areas of your life.

CHAPTER 15:

The power of habits

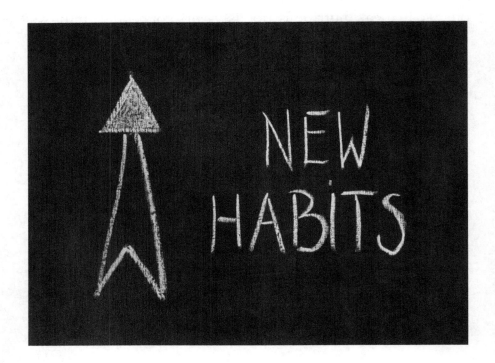

Checklist of Key Habits to Cultivate

Read through this list regularly to see if you are following these guidelines.

Visualize yourself at your ideal target weight regularly and believe it is a reality.

Repeat your affirmations daily.

Focus on your self-hypnosis techniques regularly.

Free yourself from any unpleasant habits or negative conditioning.

Do not weigh yourself or use the word diet. Do not discuss your weight with anyone. Maintain a silent, disciplined quest to improve the quality of your life.

Stick to three small, healthy major meals a day—breakfast, lunch, and dinner. Avoid eating late.

Avoid processed food and food with excess sugar, additives, or chemicals. Choose organic food when possible.

Drink fresh mineral water (that you love the taste of) between meals in place of snacking.

Always eat very slowly, chew your food thoroughly, and be fully engaged while eating. Stop eating as soon as you are full.

Be grateful for each healthy meal.

Get into the habit of moving your body as often as possible. Look for simple everyday opportunities to be active.

Exercise little and often, every day if possible, even if it is just a short walk or a mini-trampoline workout for ten minutes in the morning.

Never criticize yourself and apply the 80/20 rule.

Regularly program your mind to love your new healthy, holistic lifestyle.

Take Things Slowly

Eating should not be treated as a race. Eat slowly. This just means that you should take your time in relishing and enjoying your food, it is a healthy thing! So, how long do you have to grind up the food in your mouth? Well, there is no specific time food should be chewed, but 18-25 bites are enough to enjoy the food mindfully.

This can be hard at first, mainly if you have been used to speed eating for an exceptionally long time. Why not try some new techniques like using chopsticks when you are accustomed to spoon and fork?

Or use your non-dominant hand when eating. These strategies can slow you down and improve your awareness.

Avoid Distractions

To make things simpler for you, just make it a habit of sitting down and staying away from distractions. The handful of nuts that you eat as you walk through the kitchen and the bunch of morning snacks you nibbled while standing in front of your fridge can be hard to recall. According to researchers, people tend to eat more when they are doing other things too. You should, therefore, sit down and focus on your food to prevent mindless eating behaviors.

Savor Every Bite

Do not forget that eating mindfully is not only about enjoying the food you eat, but your health too, and without feeling guilty and uncomfortable. Relishing the sight, taste, and smell of your diet is utterly worth it. This can be so easy if you take things gradually and do not rush to perfection. Make small changes towards awareness until you are a fully mindful eater. So, eat slowly and savor the good food you are eating and the proper nutrition you give to your body.

Mind the Presentation

Regardless of how busy you are, it is good to set the table, making sure it looks divine. A lovely set of utensils, placement, and napkin made of eco-friendly cloth material is a perfect reminder that you need to sit down and pay attention when you have your meals.

Plate Your Food

Serving yourself and portioning your food before bringing the plate to the table can help you consume a modest amount, rather than putting a platter on the table from which to replenish continually. You can do this even with crackers, chips, nuts, and other snack foods.

Keep yourself away from the temptation of eating straight from a bag of chips and different types of food. It is also helpful to resize the bag or place the food in smaller containers to stay aware of the amount of food you are eating.

Having a bright idea of how much you have eaten will make you stop eating when you are full or even sooner.

Always Choose Quality over Quantity

By selecting smaller amounts of the most beautiful food within your means, you will end up enjoying and feeling satisfied without the chance of overeating.

It will be helpful if you spend time preparing your meals using quality and fresh ingredients. Cooking can be a pleasurable and relaxing experience if you only let yourself into it.

On top of this, you can achieve the peace of mind that comes from knowing what is in the food you are eating.

Do Not Invite Your Thoughts and Emotions to Dinner

Just as many other factors affect our sense of mindful eating, as well as the digestive system, it would come as no surprise that our thoughts and emotions play just as much of an important role.

It happens on the odd occasion that one comes home after a long and tiresome day and you feel somewhat "worked up," irritated and angry. This is when negative and even destructive thoughts creep in while you are having supper.

The best practice would be to avoid this altogether. Therefore, if you feel unhappy or angry in any way, go for a walk before supper, play with your children, or play with your family pet. But, whatever you do, take your mind off your negative emotions before you attempt to have a meal.

Make a Good Meal Plan for Each Week

When you start the diet, it is advised to stick to the meal plan that comes with the diet. There should be a meal plan of 2 weeks or four weeks attached to the diet's guideline. Once you are familiar with the food list, prohibited ingredients, cooking techniques, and grocery shopping for your diet, it will be easier for you to twist and change things in the meal plan. Do not try to change the meal plan for the first two weeks.

Stick to the meal plan they give you. If you try to change it right at the beginning, you may feel lost or feel terrified in the front. So, it is advised to introduce new recipes and ideas after two weeks into the diet.

Drink Lots of Water

Staying hydrated is the key to living a healthy life in general. It is not relevant for only diets, but in general, we should always be drinking enough water to keep ourselves hydrated. Dehydration can bring forth many unwanted diseases. When you are dehydrated, you feel very dizzy, lightheaded, nauseous, and lethargic. You cannot focus on anything well. Urinary infection occurs, which triggers other health issues.

Being on a diet, the purpose of drinking water is to help you process the different food you are eating and to help digest it well. Water helps in proper digestion; it helps in extracting bad minerals from our body. Water also gives us a glow on the skin.

Never Skip Breakfast

It is very essential to eat a full breakfast to keep yourself moving actively throughout the day. It gives you a significant boost, good metabolism, and your digestion starts appropriately functioning during the day. When you skip breakfast, everything sort of disrupts. Your day starts slow, and soon, you would feel restless.

It is crucial to have a good meal at the beginning of your day in order to be productive for the rest of the day.

If you are busy, try to have your breakfast on the go. Grab breakfast in a box or a mason jar and have it in the car or on the bus or whatever transport you are using to get to your work. You can also have your breakfast at a healthy restaurant where they serve food that is in sync with your diet.

Eat Protein

Protein is perfect for the body. It helps your brain function better. Protein can come from both animal and non-animal products. So even if you are a vegetable or vegan, you can still enjoy your protein from plants. Soy, mushroom, legumes, and nuts are a few examples.

Eating protein keeps you strong and healthy. Eating protein increases your brain function.

On the other hand, if you do not eat enough protein for the day, your entire way would be wasted. You will not be able to focus on anything properly. You would feel dizzy and weak all through the day. If you are a vegetarian or vegan, you can enjoy avocado, coconut, almond, cashew, soy, and mushroom to get protein.

Eat Super Foods

Most people eat foods that do not necessarily affect them in the best way. Where some foods may enhance some people's energy levels, it may impact others more negatively.

The important thing is to know your food. It may be a good idea to keep a food journal, and if you know that certain foods affect you negatively, one should try to avoid those foods and stick to healthier options.

It is a fact that most people enjoy foods which they should probably not be eating. However, if you wish to eat mindfully and enhance your health and a general sense of wellbeing, then it would be best to eat foods that will precisely do that.

There are also various foods that are classified as superfoods. These would include your lean and purest sources of protein, such as free-range chicken, as well as a variety of fresh fruit, vegetable, and herbs.

Stop Multitasking While You Eat

Multitasking is defined as the simultaneous execution of more than one activity at one time. Though it is a skill that we should master, it often leads to unproductive activity. The development of our economy leads to a more hectic way of living. Most of us develop the habit of doing one thing while doing another. This is true even when it comes to eating.

Smaller Plates, Taller Glasses

This habit changer ties in a little bit with drinking more water; however, it is a bit different. People tend to fill up their plates with food, so the size of the plate matters. If you have a large plate, you will put more food on your plate but, if you have a smaller plate, you will have less food on your plate.

Stay Positive

The secret to succeeding in anything is being optimistic. When you start something new, always stay positive regarding it. It would be best if you kept a positive mind, an open mind relatively. You cannot be anxious, hasty, and restless in a diet. You need to stay calm and do everything that calms you down. Overthinking can lead to being bored and not interested in the diet very soon. The power of positivity is immense. It cannot be compared with anything else. On the other hand, when you start something with a negative mindset, it eventually does not work out. You end up leaving it behind or failing at it because you had doubts right at the beginning. A doubtful mind cannot focus properly, and the best never comes out from a suspicious mind. Eating mindlessly can cause anyone to eat way too much, which happens to most of us. The problem is that when people are eating, they are hardly thinking about what they are doing. Instead, their minds are on other things, which leads them not to be aware of how much they are eating.

Self-discipline

What is Self-Discipline?

The term "self-discipline" is a bit of a catch-all phrase that represents a variety of different mental strengths that a person might possess. These include strengths such as restraint, perseverance, mental endurance, emotional intelligence, the ability to think before acting, the ability to finish what you started, and the strength to carry out your plans regardless of what hardships may arise on your path. When you have self-discipline, you also have self-control. You have discovered the golden ticket for avoiding unhealthy excess of anything that may lead to unwanted or negative consequences in your life, and, as a result, you find yourself achieving far greater heights of success.

Self-discipline truly is the gateway for people to move from dreaming about success to actually making success happen for themselves. When you focus on increasing your self-discipline, acting in self-disciplined ways becomes easier and easier, so, in a sense, it becomes easier for you to succeed. Now, understand that this does not mean that you will not face challenges and that your path will not be rife with hardship. You will face challenges, and things will get incredibly hard for you at various points throughout your pursuit of success. However, when you have self-discipline in your corner, arguably those challenges and hardships become less complicated because you have learned how to use your mind to help you succeed successfully. Those who have yet to increase their self-discipline find themselves using their mind against their success by allowing it to automatically come up with excuses for why they cannot create the results they desire to make in their life.

Developing self-discipline in your life does not have to be some strenuous, challenging practice that leaves you feeling like you have absolutely nothing good to look forward to. There is no reason to starve yourself from having fun, engaging in the occasional distraction, or allowing yourself to immerse yourself in your comfort zone for some time. The difference is that you are not doing these activities to stay comfortable, but instead, you are engaging in them mindfully and with the ability to stop engaging in them when you need to employ your mind for something different, such as achieving growth in any given area of your life. When you are self-disciplined, these behaviors become leisurely behaviors as they are meant to be, rather than default behaviors that prevent you from ever getting ahead in life.

Most people who pursue self-discipline agree that it is quite challenging at first, but as they begin to get the hang of it, their self-discipline becomes more enjoyable. In fact, they even start to look forward to engaging in self-discipline because it can be so fun to live a life where you are entirely in control of your actions, your impulses, and your urges, and you are capable of doing everything with great intention. Through this, you become your own most remarkable tool in your success, and, as a result, you achieve far more.

Trying to fight against your low mental toughness would be like trying to lift a 400lb weight when you have never weight trained before. It would be ludicrous to believe that you could do so consistently without seriously hurting yourself.

Likewise, there is no way that you can push against mental resistance when you lack the toughness to do so. Building your mental toughness by building your self-discipline will directly equip you with the strength you need to do all of the heavy liftings in your life and get yourself to the level of success you desire.

Why is Self-Discipline So Important?

Sure, you know that self-discipline is the number one key to success and that without it, you are going to struggle massively when it comes to achieving anything. But why is self-discipline so necessary? I mean, why can you not be successful unless you have this skill in your life?

The answer to this is simple: self-discipline is what is going to directly drive you through any challenge or setback you face in your life, especially on the path to achieving your goals.

The power of faith

Are you determined to lose weight? You want to prevent heart disease complications, diabetes, and elevated cholesterol levels associated with being overweight for most individuals, including yourself. However, because of their fitness, not everyone goes on a quest to lose weight. You can want to lose weight because you see weight loss as a way to make others look desirable and improve your self-image. To recover your usual body weight, there are several preventive steps you might take. People worldwide spend thousands and even millions of dollars annually on losing weight by attempting these steps. Exercise gadgets, healthier organic foods, dietary supplements, slimming pills, diets, and fitness clubs are spent on these vast amounts of money every day.

That simple little secret of weight loss is the magic response. You must change the way you think about yourself and your food. Take this case: do you recall those times, when you were on that expensive wonder diet, that you watched your weight rigorously but still struggled to keep your eyes off that creamy dessert after meals or didn't even feel bold enough to cut off your chocolate craving?

It may not be as easy for you to believe, but I can assure you that the reason you feel you're losing the war is easy. The explanation is that you have not changed the habits of your old thoughts about how you felt about the creamy dessert and the chocolate bar and, more importantly, about yourself. This example is to show you that your thinking patterns can influence your weight loss.

As human beings, our emotions and beliefs affect our actions, which then cause us to respond in a certain way to a situation. The little thoughts you used to have about the beautiful dessert or chocolate after your meals would have prompted you to choose to skip the dessert or just take a bite and then finish it all. Unfortunately, your above intervention will be to the detriment of your effort at losing any weight.

You may also regulate your emotions, on the other hand, or make suggestions in your mind to alter how you feel about the dessert and chocolate. The good news is that you can control your emotions or make suggestions to your mind on how you react to the dessert or the pudding without weakening your weight loss program. Hypnosis will show you how you can make these suggestions to control the emotions in the head.

Hypnosis is an interaction between yourself and the hypnotist. A hypnotist is someone who is trained to use hypnotic methods or therapy and is skilled. The hypnotist will attempt to manipulate or make suggestions on your thoughts and behavior during this interaction by specifically focusing on ideas and images that may elicit any expected results verbally.

You can receive advice from the hypnotist to lose weight through Hypnosis that will change your previous emotions or perceptions about the factors that could have contributed to your weight gain. You may also opt not to see the hypnotist face to face when you chose to use Hypnosis.

In addition to this being the overview of the mechanism of helping to facilitate progress, it also happens to be a mechanism that many of us have found works naturally. Some of us have come upon the process of programming our minds with our ambitions and accomplishments, and milestones we aspire to and have been able to proceed and accomplish them.

CHAPTER 16:

Reprogram your mind

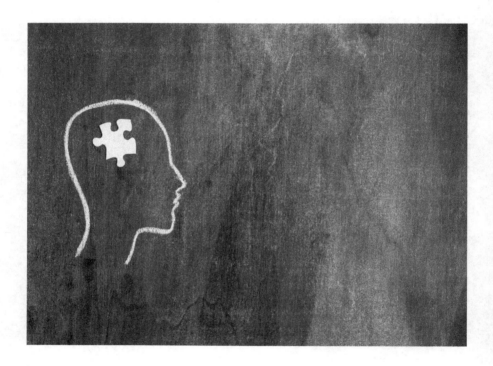

D o you remember the first time you learned to do something new, for example, drive a new car? You may have driven for years but learning all about an unfamiliar vehicle can be frustrating. How do you turn on the lights or the windshield wipers? Is the gas tank filled from the left or right side? Programming the clock and radio for the first time can take a while. The first trip or two can be difficult. But then you learn where everything is and how it all works, and the mechanics become almost an automatic, unconscious process.

You can use that same inherent learning ability to teach yourself to love exercising and healthy food. You can learn to love feeling fit and healthy and to find fattening food repulsive. Whatever your weight loss aims, you can reprogram your mind in specific ways to help you achieve your goals. Learning these new habits is a matter of repetition.

The more you visualize and absorb these affirmations, the quicker you create the new inner belief. It is also gratifying because you will create very relaxing mental states that benefit your general health and well-being.

How Affirmations Work

A goal is a specific target that you set for yourself to achieve within a fixed time frame. An affirmation is a statement of intent that you repeat to yourself repeatedly. Affirmations need to be phrases and phrases said clearly and concisely with a slight emphasis. Whenever you use your claims, feel as though you are drawing the words inside you, as though you are teaching the inner part of yourself a new belief. You must always state affirmations in the present tense and focus on them as if they are a reality now. You must decide the wording of your affirmations upon before you begin a self-hypnosis session, and you must work on only one goal at a time. For example, don't work on releasing fear and losing weight in the same session. While you can use several affirmations in one session, they must all relate to the one chosen goal for that session. You must make affirmations completely unambiguous and always accentuate the positive. I use the words "I love to ..." to start many of my affirmations because love is a useful, emotive phrase, and I find this confirmation has a profound impact.

Writing your goals and affirmations is very important because it gives words power and meaning, reminding you constantly of where you are heading. It also spells out your intent loud and clear, adding clarity to your aims and helping to compound your new belief structures.

Bringing Yourself Back to Full Consciousness

If you practice this process before going to sleep, you need not count up from one to ten. Before you begin your consultation, just tell yourself that the trance will become a deep, natural sleep from which you may wake within the morning feeling nice and refreshed.

Think of the analogy of reprogramming a computer with new data. What you put into it will come back out. Totally immerse yourself in your aims. When you are in a trance, use all of your senses to compound the phrases and make your affirmations and visualizations colorful and real. Do not worry if you are not good at visualizing; you may have a different dominant sense. Most people are visual, but others absorb information more easily through another sense—feeling, hearing, smell, or even taste. That is why it is vital to use all of your senses when visualizing so that your more dominant understanding will help you absorb the new beliefs at a deeper level.

The Power of Your Mind

Never underestimate the power you have inside you. Your mind has incredible potential. All around the world, there are stories of human beings achieving impossible feats. There are documented instances of moms being able to summon superhuman strength to lift a vehicle off the floor to keep their youngsters trapped underneath.

When the mother sees her baby in a hazard, she doesn't prevent and think; I can't elevate that vehicle because it weighs too much. The handiest concept in her thoughts is to save her toddler; the truth that the car is too heavy to raise does not enter her thinking. This is the vital thing to how she will do it—there isn't a doubt in her mind, and she is entirely focused on lifting the automobile. Through excessive awareness and sheer force of will, the mom can summon the electricity to boost an automobile weighing greater than a ton.

The survival instinct is the most effective driver humans possess, and while this is threatened, in extreme circumstances, we can do matters that defy logic. When we're at serious risk, our focus turns heightened, and we enter an altered country of consciousness. In this modified nation, we can use exceptional strength and electricity.

By using self-hypnosis, you may engage your thoughts similarly and reap so much. Think of the tale of the mom lifting the automobile as a metaphor for your fitness journey. Never put a limit on what you may do. You can reap, in reality, something while you discover ways to the awareness of your thoughts.

CHAPTER 17:

The importance of having goals

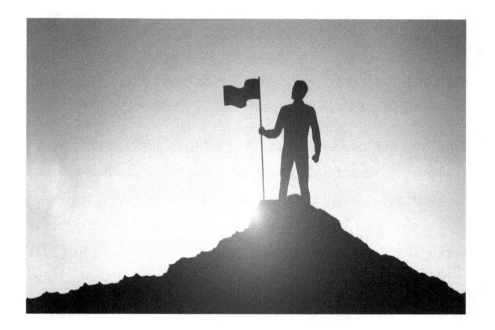

I t's a good idea to grab a food journal to track you're eating on a day-to-day basis, so you are practicing awareness of what you are eating. This helps you consciously process what you are about to put into your mouth or reflect on what you already ate on any given day. It's been shown that when you are more conscious of your choices, you make better ones.

It is essential to be realistic about your goals, and you must discuss this with your surgeon. I also need to note here; for some individuals, the BMI chart can be deceiving.

This does not mean you get a free pass to bypass the BMI chart. However, it's essential to see where you fall and whether it's a factor in your actual body fat percentage overall. As someone who is 5'11 tall, I know I'm never going to be 160lbs, and that is precisely what the chart shows I should be. I'm not saying that you should hide your head in the sand or state you're 'big-boned' if you're not.

The goal is for you to lose weight and to be healthy for your body's height. It's all about proportion. The goal here is NOT to get you down to a specific weight per se, but to get you to a weight that YOU are comfortable at, and at a weight and size in which you feel good living in your body. You, feeling comfortable in your own body, makes all the difference.

Let's look at your personal goals for the short-term and long-term to help you understand where you want to be.

What are the realistic goals for your weight and height?

How much do you expect to lose overall?

What is your height?

What was your highest weight?

What was your Surgery Weight?

What is your Current Weight?

What is your ideal ending Goal Weight?

What are your post-surgery (pounds lost) goals for:

Month 1:

What size do you want to be in?

How do you want to feel?

Month 3:

What size do you want to be in?

How do you want to feel?

Month 6:

What size do you want to be in?

How do you want to feel?

Month 9:

What size do you want to be in?

How do you want to feel?

Month 12:

What size do you want to be in?

How do you want to feel?

Month 18:

What size do you want to be in?

How do you want to feel?

Month 24:

What size do you want to be in?

How do you want to feel?

Month 30:

What size do you want to be in?

How do you want to feel?

Month 36:

What size do you want to be in?

How do you want to feel?

If you don't know what you want, how will you go after it?

Clarity is so important. Knowing what you want is step one. If you do not yet know what you will do once you lose the weight, start thinking about it now.

The plan is to lose weight and to do all the things you have not had the opportunity to do as an obese individual. There's so much more life for you to live and many things I know you want to do.

Do you have a desire to travel to Europe and walk through the ancient streets of Rome?

Do you want to walk/run a 5k?

Do you want to chase after your grandchildren and be able to pick them up at a moment's notice?

Or would you like to feel comfortable making love to your husband/wife?

What is it that means the most to you?

What are those things that you're excited to do now that you're losing weight?

List them out.

CHAPTER 18:

Step-by-Step Hypnotherapy for Weight Loss

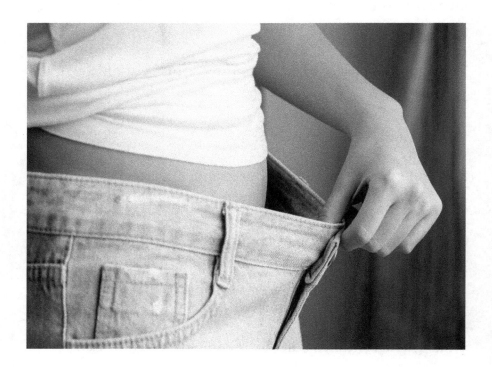

I f you don't figure entrancing will enable you to change your emotions, it will probably have little impact.

Become agreeable. Go to a spot where you may not be stressed. This can resemble your bed, a couch, or a pleasant, comfortable chair anyplace. Ensure you bolster your head and neck. Wear loose garments and ensure the temperature is set at an agreeable level. It might be simpler to unwind if you play some delicate music while mesmerizing yourself, particularly something instrumental.

Focus on an item. Discover something to take a gander at and focus on in the room, ideally something somewhat above you. Utilize your concentration for clearing your leader of all contemplations on this item. Make this article the main thing that you know about.

Breathing is crucial. When you close your eyes, inhale profoundly. Reveal to yourself the greatness of your eyelids and let them fall delicately. Inhale profoundly with an ordinary mood as your eyes close. Concentrate on your breathing, enabling it to assume control over your whole personality, much like the item you've been taking a gander at previously. Feel progressively loose with each fresh breath. Envision that your muscles disperse all the pressure and stress. Permit this inclination from your face, your chest, your arms, lastly, your legs to descend your body.

When you're entirely loose, your psyche should be clear, and you will be a self-mesmerizing piece.

Display a pendulum. Customarily, the development of a pendulum moving to and from has been utilized to energize the center is spellbinding. Picture this pendulum in your psyche, driving to and from. Concentrate on it as you unwind to help clear your brain.

Start by focusing on 10 to 1 in your mind. You advise yourself as you check down that you are steadily getting further into entrancing. State, "10, I'm alleviating. 9, I get increasingly loose. 8. I can feel my body spreading, unwinding. 7, Nothing yet unwinding I can handle.... 1, I'm resting profoundly. Keep in mind that you will be in a condition of spellbinding when you accomplish one all through.

Waking up from self-hypnosis. Once during spellbinding, you have accomplished what you need, you should wake up. From 1 to 10, check back. State in your mind: "1, I wake up. 2, I'll feel like I woke up from a significant rest when I tally down. 3, I feel wakeful more.... 10, I'm wakeful, I'm new.

Develop a plan. Reinventing your mind with spellbinding requires consistent redundancy. You ought to endeavor in a condition of spellbinding to go through around twenty minutes per day. While beneath, shift back and forth between portions of the underneath referenced methodologies. Attempt to assault your poor eating rehearses from any edge.

Learn to refrain from emotional overeating. One of the main things you should endeavor to do under mesmerizing is to influence yourself. You are not intrigued by the frightful nibble of food you experience issues kicking. Pick something that you will, in general, revel in, like frozen yogurt. State, "Dessert tastes poor and makes me feel debilitated." Repeat twenty minutes until you're prepared to wake up from the trance. Keep in mind; excellent eating regimen doesn't suggest you have to quit eating; simply eat less awful sustenance. Simply influence yourself to devour less food, you know, is undesirable.

Write your very own positive mantra. Self-spellbinding ought to likewise be utilized to reinforce your longing to eat better. Compose a mantra to rehash in a trance state. It harms me and my body when I overeat.

Imagine the best thing for you. Picture what you might want to be more beneficial to support your longing to live better. From when you were more slender, take a picture of yourself or do your most extreme to figure what you'd resemble in the wake of shedding pounds. Concentrate on this image under mesmerizing. Envision the trust you'd feel on the off chance that you'd be more advantageous. This will cause you to comprehend that when you wake up. Eat each supper with protein. Protein is especially valuable at topping you off and can improve your digestion since it advances muscle improvement. Fish, lean meat, eggs, yogurt, nuts, and beans are great wellsprings of protein. A steak each dinner might be counterproductive, yet in case you're eager, eating on nuts could go far to helping you accomplish your objectives.

Eat a few modest meals daily. If you don't eat for quite a while, your digestion will go down, and you will stop fat consumption. If you expend something modest once every three or four hours, your metabolism will go up, and when you plunk down for dinner, you will be less hungry.

Eat organically grown foods. You will be loaded up with foods grown from the ground and furnish you with supplements without putting any pounds on. To start shedding pounds, nibble on bananas rather than treats to quicken weight reduction.

Cut down on unhealthy fats. It tends to be helpful for you to have unsaturated fats, similar to those in olive oil. Nonetheless, you should endeavor to limit your saturated fat and trans-fat intake. Both of these are significant factors that add to coronary illness.

Learn more about healthy cooking. In preparing meals, trans fats are common, mainly when eating meals, sweets, and fast food.

Saturated fats may not be as bad as trans fats. However, they might be undesirable. Primary saturated fat sources include spreads, cheddar cheese, grease, red meat, and milk. The journey to weight loss is not an easy one. A person needs a lot of help and motivation to succeed. With the use of hypnotherapy, one can easily stay the course and watch the pounds melt away. Following the guide above and with a credible hypnotherapist or mastering self-hypnosis will help you achieve your goals.

The Benefits of Hypnotherapy for Losing Weight

Hypnotherapy that is geared towards helping you lose weight can help you develop a more positive image. The session usually starts with accepting your situation and doing something about it, not because of the pressure of society but because of health reasons.

Hypnosis will reframe your mind and will help you better understand you're "why" or the reason behind your goal for weight loss. This alternative session will help you manage your weight because it directly taps your motives and self-interest.

Another benefit of hypnotherapy for weight loss is it can help you relieve stress. The meditative component of Hypnosis can help you achieve a calmer and more relaxed mind. Relieving stress is important in weight loss as studies show the connection between stress and an increase in appetite.

Hypnotherapy will also rewire your conscious and subconscious mind so you can feel good about exercise and healthy diets. These two components go hand in hand in weight loss, and through Hypnosis, you will see them as allies and not as a burden.

The Downsides of Hypnotherapy for Weight Loss

Like other weight-loss treatments, hypnotherapy also has its disadvantages, albeit these are minor and tolerable ones.

Using Hypnosis to combat obesity is not invasive and usually works well with other treatments for losing weight. You also don't need to take any pills or supplements for the medicine to become effective.

One major downside of hypnotherapy is that it may not work for everyone. According to a Stanford study, 25% of the global population simply can't be placed under Hypnosis, mainly because their brains are wired. This treatment requires the patient to be willing. So, if you feel forced to do it, it may not work for you.

Another downside of using hypnotherapy for weight loss is the price. The cost of a hypnotherapy session per hour may vary depending on where you live, but the range is between $75 and $300 an hour for a session with a professional hypnotherapist.

So, if you get into a session at least once a week or more in a month, it can add up quickly. In addition, most insurance companies will not cover hypnotherapy, so you may have to pay for the sessions from your pocket. But if it is approved as a component of a mental health package, you might be covered, so be sure to check with your insurance provider.

CHAPTER 19:

Lose weight fast and naturally
with Hypnosis

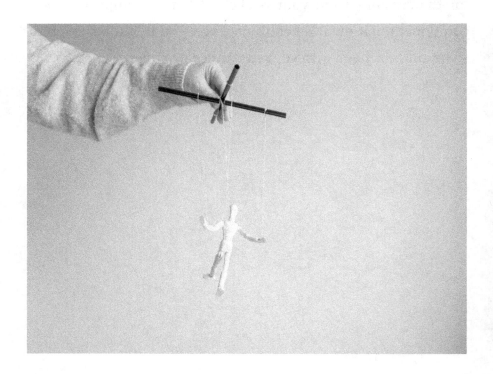

First, start by placing your hand on your stomach. As you do this, feel the body that exists underneath. It's not the one you want right now, but it's the one that you have. As you breathe in, feel your stomach expand.

As you let that air out, feel your stomach flatten. Now, count to five with me as you breathe in. One, two, three, four, five. Count to six as you breathe out. Hold for an extra second because I want you to feel your stomach flatten. Become aware of how different your body can change.

Now, sit with your hands somewhere comfortable, focusing only on your closed eyes. Again, keep breathing in and out, noticing the differences that you can feel in your body through your stomach muscles. The things that our bodies are capable of are pretty incredible. Knowing all the abilities, we have with them can be very enlightening.

When we are in tune with our bodies and attached to all of the things they can do, it's going to be much easier to make sure that we are making healthy decisions that are best for them.

Now, slowly let your mind drift somewhere relaxing. Pick a place in nature. Maybe it's a forest, a beach, or a large grassy field. Wherever it is, I want you to envision this. Now, I'm going to count to ten again, and as I do, your mind is going black. One, two three, four, five, six, seven, eight, nine, ten.

Now, you see nothing but black. As you focus on nothing, a small light emerges, and you see it starting to grow. As it does, you become more relaxed, still feeling the air enter and exit your body. The light keeps going, and before you know it, it is pouring all over your body.

You suddenly realize that you aren't thinking about this place in nature; you are there. As you look around, there is green surrounding you. The blue sky emerges through the leafy green trees, and you can feel the warm sun start to warm your skin.

A cool breeze comes over your body, and you feel the freshness through your hair. You are not afraid of being alone in this place in nature. It is something that you have been waiting for. This is what you deserve.

You start to walk forward, not going anywhere in particular. As you take each step, you begin to see a small building in the distance. You are slowly walking, feeling your body relax. You feel light, fresh, healthy. Something about the way you feel now is different than how you did before.

The building is right in front of you now, and you take it upon yourself to walk in. as you open the door, light pours onto you, and you suddenly feel even more rejuvenated. The building is air-conditioned, and you can tell that it is fresh and new. You aren't sure where you are, but it doesn't matter. No one seems to be there, but you are not afraid to be alone. As you walk in, you see a mirror standing right in front of you.

At first, you are afraid to look into it. There might be a person looking back at you that you do not want to see. Something is telling you that it is time to look into this mirror, however. As you walk up to it, you are shocked to see the person looking back at you. This is a person that you don't recognize at first. They are healthy. They are smiling. Their skin is clear, and their hair is radiant. They are fit, and you can tell that they are working out. The more you look at them, the more you realize that this is you. This is the version that you have been waiting for.

You have had visions in the past of what it might look like if you were to decide to go through with your weight loss journey finally. Now, you are here. You are looking into the mirror and seeing a person that you have been hoping for all along. You are happy and healthy. You are confident, and you are excited.

As you look into the mirror, you suddenly remember all that it took to get there. There were moments where you thought that you couldn't do it. There were times when the only thing that felt right was for you to give up. There were many obstacles in your way, but you finally dared to fight through them and get what you wanted.

As you look at your legs, you see that they are healthy. They carried you for your entire life, helping you get places that you would never have imagined. You can see the outline of your muscles in them, so strong and sleek. As you move up, you see the flat stomach that you have always wanted.

You might still have a few stretch marks, but they are there as a reminder of how much you worked for your health. You fought for yourself for your body. You went through things that others aren't able to do on their own. You see this in your torso. All the food that looked so appetizing that you said "no" to shows in your flat stomach now. Every time you chose something healthy instead of something simply tasty is making itself present in your body.

As you look into the mirror, you see that your chest is strong as well. This healthy chest protects your heart, and you can feel it working well as it sends blood throughout your body. You are feeling energized, correct, fulfilled, and happy. Finally, you see your shoulders and arms. These are so strong and have also helped to carry you so far.

You look at them from your fingers to your neck, toned and supporting the rest of your body. Though you have seen all of the important changes throughout your body, the most important thing is how large your smile is now. Your cheeks are stretched to show the radiance that has always existed inside of you and can finally be present now.

It feels so good to know that you look this good, but what is even better than that is that you are so comfortable with your body.

Throughout your weight loss, you learned how to take care of yourself in a healthy way so that you will be able to keep the weight off for a long time. There were moments when all you wanted was a specific body, but right here, smiling into the mirror, you know now that the most important thing is that you are happy.

It is time now for me to bring you out of the Hypnosis. When I count to ten, you will be back into the present world, ready to start your journey. One, two, three, four, five, six, seven, eight, nine, ten.

Using Hypnosis to Overcome the Mental Barriers

We create habit patterns through repetition, and with time, they become automatic responses to the environment.

Deep in our minds, we have strong ideas that keep us thinking of unhealthy behaviors. Over time, people train the mind to believe that unhealthy behaviors, like emotional eating or overindulging, are necessary to maintain our well-being. And as such, if the mind repeatedly thinks of these behaviors, long-term changes become very difficult.

Emotional eating is just an example of associations that negatively affect our efforts to lose weight.

There are several other associations that people develop, which impact their relationship with food negatively. Some of these associations that hinder weight loss include:

- Food and constant eating help in distracting us from anxiety, anger, and sadness

- Food is a comforting tool; it comforts us when we are feeling sad or stressed

- Overeating sugary or unhealthy foods are associated with good times and celebrations

- Sugary and unhealthy foods are a reward

- Overeating can help one to overcome the fear that you won't manage to lose weight

- Food is a source of entertainment when one is feeling bored

Ultimately, losing weight successfully with Hypnosis requires that we assess these root causes, understand them, and finally reframe them.

This is what Hypnosis can do!

Reframing Your Addiction to Food using Hypnosis

The first step of a hypnosis process is: To identify why you have not achieved your weight loss goals. How does this happen? To understand your shortfalls, a hypnotherapist will typically ask you questions about your eating behaviors and your weight loss journey. This information gathering process will help you identify what you might need to change to attain your goal.

After understanding your eating habits, a hypnotherapist will guide you through an induction process, which entails the relaxation of the mind and body. You will enter a hypnotic state. While in the state, your mind will become highly suggestible; you will have shed off your conscious, critical mind, allowing the hypnotherapist to speak directly to your unconscious mind.

In Hypnosis, you will be provided with positive affirmations and suggestions, and you may be asked to visualize changes. There are several positive suggestions for rapid weight loss, including:

Identify the possible unconscious eating habits—With Hypnosis, you will identify the negative unconscious eating patterns that you have developed over time. When you are hypnotized, you can become more aware of what makes you consume unhealthy food and develop strategies to change the habit.

Reframing your inner voice— with Hypnosis, you will be able to "speak" with the inner voice that misleads you to eat unhealthy food. A hypnotherapist can help you "communicate" with your inner voice. Still, he/she can also turn your inner voice into a support system that guides you to consider positive and rational suggestions.

Developing healthy coping tactics—with Hypnosis, you will develop healthy ways to cope with stress. During Hypnosis, you will become aware that snacking is not the only way to deal with anxiety and stress. You will, therefore, consider other coping strategies.

Improve your food choices— you might be addicted to junk food, but you will develop a low for healthier foods with Hypnosis.

Encouraging healthy eating— With Hypnosis, you will develop the habit of choosing healthier eating habits such as reducing your food portion sizes or rehearsing certain eating choices like taking the remaining food home when you are eating in a restaurant.

Visualizing success— a hypnotic program will encourage you to visualize how you can achieve weight loss goals. Once you visualize how it feels to lose weight, you will have higher chances of practicing the weight-loss tactics.

Improve your confidence— with Hypnosis, and you will develop positive suggestions that boost your self-confidence. With confidence, you will be able to achieve your weight loss goals.

Identifying the unconscious indicators— with hypnotic therapy, you will identify the signals you receive from your body. This can help you understand when you are full and identify the difference between feeling hungry and being thirsty.

When doing Hypnosis, these suggestions can help you to overcome your cravings and poor eating habits. Not all of them apply to every person. However, the goal is to develop a hypnosis plan, which includes the only relevant suggestions.

How Hypnosis helps you Achieve Rapid Weight Loss

During Hypnosis, your mind becomes open to any suggestions. Studies have shown that your brain is likely to experience interesting changes when in the hypnotic state, allowing learning about the information you are receiving without having to think critically or consciously.

In this state, you are always detached from your conscious mind. Thus, you don't interrupt your thoughts with a question about what you are hearing. And this is how Hypnosis helps break down barriers that prevent you from shedding off weight.

In hypnotherapy, repetition is the key to success. This explains why many hypnotherapists provide you with self-hypnosis recordings, which you own to listen to repeatedly.

The brain's barriers are always very strong, and only through repeated Hypnosis can you untangle yourself from the convictions.

Hypnosis teaches the mind how to think differently about eating and food. The suggestions we discussed above can help you achieve the following:

Control Food Cravings

Weight loss hypnotic techniques can help you to detach yourself from cravings and isolate yourself from unhealthy foods. For instance, during Hypnosis, you might be asked to visualize how you will send away the cravings. Suggestions can help in reframing cravings and teach you how to manage them efficiently.

Success

Expectations of an individual dictate his/her reality. With the expectation of success, we are apt to take the steps necessary to attain success.

Hypnosis can plant this seed of success in your mind, thus, giving you the unconscious power to keep yourself on course.

Positivity

Nobody likes negativity, and our brains are no different. Negative thoughts can spoil your ability and dedication to lose weight.

Through Hypnosis, you will become aware of the foods that you "can't eat." These foods do not help your body or health in any way. Thus, hypnotherapy will make you understand that you are not punishing yourself by abstaining from these foods, but you improve your overall being.

Preparing for Relapse

Our minds have been trained to think that relapsing from a journey or goal is a sinful act, as it is a reason to give up. However, Hypnosis gives us the chance of relapsing differently. The relapse becomes an opportunity to examine what went wrong, learn from it, and then prepare for future temptation.

Modifying Behaviors

We can only achieve big goals by taking small steps at a time. Hypnosis empowers us to take the step for these small changes, which eventually result in bigger goals.

For instance, when you always reward yourself with high-calorie content and sugary foods, you will, over time, choose a healthier reward through Hypnosis.

Visualizing Success

Hypnosis is considered a powerful motivator. You might be able to visualize your future-self, telling others how easy it is to lose weight.

Getting Started with Weight Loss Hypnosis

Do you want to start your weight loss journey today? To begin with, you have several different options. One of the options is to visit a certified hypnotherapist who will offer you face-to-face hypnosis sessions. Alternatively, you may schedule a session with a hypnotherapist via a virtual conference. Also, you may consider recorded Hypnosis for self-training. The three common hypnosis options include:

One-on-one hypnosis session

This session helps you to identify the unconscious mental barriers that may hinder you from reaching your goal. Once you acknowledge your obstacles, you will be able to develop effective strategies to overcome them. Below are the things that happen during one-on-one Hypnosis for weight loss: The hypnotherapist will guide you into reaching a state of Hypnosis or deep relaxation. Once you feel fully relaxed, the therapist will be able to access your unconscious mind, including your survival mechanisms and innate instincts.

The hypnotherapist will then use soothing, worded scripts to explore your reasons for overeating and suggest new thinking strategies through visualization. The process enables you to control any of the therapist's suggestions that you are no happy.

Guided hypnosis sessions

This hypnosis technique entails hypnosis sessions that give you the advantage of mobility. You will start the sessions whenever you are ready and always use them when you are on vacation or at home. The recorded sessions can take you through weight loss, including suggestions that are valuable to you.

Self-conducted hypnosis sessions—An advantage of this option is that it is free of charge. The main disadvantage of this approach is that it can be confusing because you may not be aware of what you are doing in the process; thus, you may not meet your weight loss goals.

CHAPTER 20:

Weight loss meditation

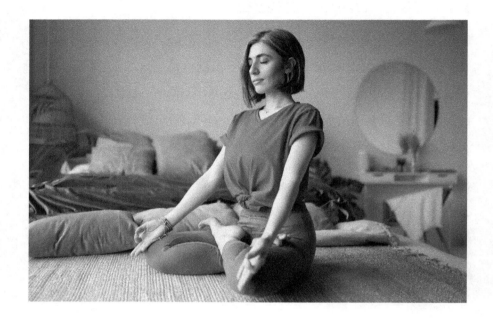

Daily Weight Loss Meditation

Meditation is in fashion. As soon as you tell someone that you have a problem, it is a rare occasion when they do not recommend you practice it. It does not matter if the problem is mental or physical.

Sometimes, people's insistence leads us to reject a plan idea. However, would it not be more interesting to ask why so many people agree to advise you the same thing?

Interest in Eastern cultures brought the influence of ideas to the forefront. And they are our existence's nucleus. Nutrition and physical exercise promote our body's optimal working.

Yet, it is also true that when our emotions aren't controlled, the brain secretes substances that affect our bodies and minds.

Therefore, physical sufferings or thoughts that make life difficult for us can appear. In this way, meditation helps to keep us safe.

Meditation lowered inflammation levels

Beyond what happened in mind, they find an inflammation measure lower than before the investigation. It indicates that perception benefits go beyond what would appear.

The group manager warns that the exact extent of its benefits cannot yet be defined. Nevertheless, the observation is adequate to multiply scientists' efforts in this regard.

It is no longer about Buddhist experiences or self-help customers who can't control.

We have evidence. However, intentional meditation enhances our quality of life. Furthermore, its effects last four months mean that it is a long-term practice that benefits us.

Given the number of harmful elements to which we are exposed, it seems reasonable to bet on this option without being able to do anything.

All this shows us how the first step to improving our health is to listen to our bodies.

It is improbable that the effects you notice when introducing a new habit constitute a mere imagination. Therefore, from here, we want to thank the efforts of many people who have defended an alternative lifestyle—another class of medicine.

Even when they have been treated as "enlightened" and a little sane, their constancy and the defense of their values have been translated into a scientific study that has proved them right and from which we will all benefit.

Practicing anti-stress meditation at home

We know that sometimes it costs. How to combine our daily obligations with that moment of anti-stress meditation? We get up with things to do and arrive at bed with a mind full of those tasks and commitments that must be fulfilled for the following day.

Be careful if the preceding paragraph is an example of what you always live in your day today. You must know how to organize times and set limits, control all those pressures that do not allow you to get rest. Ideally, you learn to balance your life. Where you are always the priority of taking care of your health and emotions, stress can hurt you a lot, and you should see it as an enemy to dominate and do small to handle it properly. We explain how to practice anti-stress meditation.

Emotional agenda

Do you keep a plan in your day to day of the things you should do? Of your obligations, appointments, meetings, appointments with teachers of children, or your visit to the doctor?

Do the same with your emotions, with your personal needs. Spend at least one hour or two hours for yourself each day. To do what you like, to be alone, and to practice anti-stress meditation. Your emotions have priority; make a hole in your day today. You deserve it, and you need it.

A moment of tranquility

It doesn't matter where it is. In your room, in the kitchen or a park.

You must be calm and surrounded by an environment that is pleasant, peaceful, and comforting. If you want, put on the music that you like, but you must be alone.

Regulate your breathing

Let's now take care of our breathing. Once you are comfortable, start to take a deep breath through your nose.

Allow your chest to swell, then let this air out little by little through your mouth.

If you repeat it six or seven times, you will begin to notice a pleasant tingling through your body, and you feel better and calmer.

Focus thoughts

What will we do after? Visualize those pressures that concern you most. Are you pressured at work? Do you have problems with your partner?

Visualize those images and keep breathing. The tension should soften, the nerves should lose their intensity, and the fear will ease. You will feel better little by little.

Positive images

Once you have focused on those images, what more pressure they cause on your being? Let's now visualize pleasant things and aspects that you would like to be living, which would make you happy.

They must be simple things: a walk on the beach; you are touching the bark of a tree, you walk through a quiet city where the sun illuminates your face and where the rumor of nearby coffee shops envelops you with a pleasant smell of coffee. Easy things make you happy. Visualize it and keep breathing deeply.

The silence

Now we close our eyes. At least for two minutes. Try not to think about anything; just let the silence envelop you. You are at peace, and you are well; there is no pressure. There are only you and a peaceful world where there are no pressures and threats, and everything is warm and pleasant.

Open your eyes in a renewed way

It is time to open your eyes and breathe normally again. Look around without moving, without getting up. Don't do it, or you'll run the risk of getting dizzy. Allow about five minutes to pass before you walk again. Indeed you feel much better, lighter, and without any pressure on your body.

New perspectives

Now that you feel more relaxed try to think about what you can do to find yourself better day by day.

Being a little happier sometimes requires that we have to make small changes. And the good thing about anti-stress meditation is that it is slowly changing us inside.

It requires us to make small changes to find the balance so that the body and the mind feel in tune again, and the pressures, the anxieties go out of our body like the smoke that escapes through a window.

Simple Meditation Exercises

Stress accumulates like oil. Paradoxically, as one increases, the other declines. Therefore, stress and energy can fuel a wide variety of sources.

For example, stress may feed on problems in various places or simply a life pattern marked by a lack of breaks. We will present simple meditation exercises to help relieve this stress.

Indeed, meditation encourages self-awareness. It is an ancient Indian peculiar millennial technique, popular in Buddhist and Hindu beliefs. It's become common in the West in recent years.

Focus your attention on breathing

The first of the simple meditation exercises is also one of the easiest to incorporate into our routine. We will do it more easily if we can adopt a relaxed position with semi-open eyes.

It is also good to focus on our breathing without trying to vary the parameters. It's about perceiving the air coming in and going out. At this moment, it is common to be distracted by different thoughts. Our mission will be to ignore them until they lose their strength.

Countdown

This technique is straightforward and is of great use when it comes to meditating. With your eyes closed, count back from high numbers such as 50 or 100 until you reach zero. The goal of this practice is to focus our attention on a single thought/activity. In this way, we will be able to eliminate the sensations produced by the rest of the stimulations.

Scan our own body

This is the most interesting one of many and simple meditation exercises. We only need to reassess the different parts of our body. For this, it is recommended to place ourselves in a place of weak stimulation. Then we will focus our attention on all parts of our body, starting from the head to finish with the feet.

We can contract and release the different muscle groups to become aware of their presence and their movement. It is a rather attractive way to observe ourselves and perceive in detail the sensations of our body.

Observe dynamically

This exercise is focused on studying our climate. Let's start with a comfortable position; the best is sitting with your eyes closed. We'll then open them to approach them for a moment. Before that, we'll have to focus on what's learned.

We'll be able to think about the various sensations that we're generating the stimulations that came to us. We may list them; think of each object's shapes and colors, or name. Furthermore, it might be an excellent way to experience our home differently if we know this at home.

Meditating in motion

Another basic meditation exercise we can put into action is based on our body's feedback of fun stimuli as it moves. For this, interaction with nature is recommended.

For example, we can take a few steps on the beach or in the woods and enjoy the warmth of the sun on our faces, the wind caresses, or the touch of plants and water on our hands. It can also be another way to make a personal observation, thinking about our body's movements as we walk.

Meditate with fire

Finally, we can use fire as a symbolic purification item to focus our meditation. We may concentrate on a campfire in nature or something simpler: a candle's flame. It will allow us to experience the heat sensations associated with fire and the shadows reflecting on the surrounding objects.

On the other side, we can list and burn negative items in our everyday lives. This positive gesture that can be performed symbolically or factually helps us free ourselves from our worries of something we have no influence over.

CHAPTER 21:

Strategies for weight loss

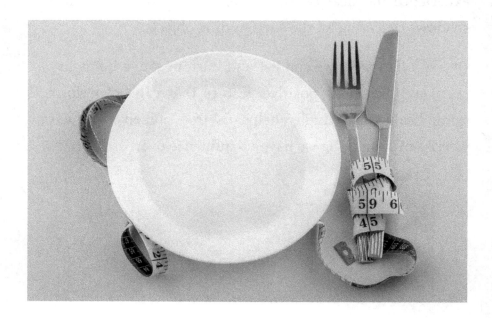

Keep a Journal

K eeping a journey is a healthy habit for many people, no matter their goals, but it's essential for someone that wants to lose weight. By writing down your different portion measurements and exercise habits, you can better ensure that you'll have a basis for evaluation. When this is done, you can predict future problems that might keep you from your goals by looking back on the days of recorded mistakes or slipups. You can see what kinds of schedules and structures aren't working to create better habits in the end. The more extensive your journaling, the better you'll be able to create your research study of your weight-loss journey, meaning you can share your progress or use it as a structure for future diets.

Avoid the Scale

The biggest issue with weight-loss strugglers comes when they see the number on the scale. Someone that wants to lose ten pounds might get discouraged if they find they only lost nine. Sometimes, people might even have to gain weight before they end up losing a pound. By avoiding the scale altogether, certain failures and disappointments can be avoided as well.

Find a different way to track your progress. You can have monthly weigh-ins, but it shouldn't be something that should be checked once a day.

Our weight fluctuates so much throughout our journey that it isn't worth stressing daily. Any checking that happens more than once a day is also likely a bad habit; you're using it to distract yourself from a bigger issue.

The Calorie Myth

When many people diet, they focus too much on calories. They'll see that a specific snack pack only has a hundred calories, which means that it's good for you, right? Wrong. When we focus too much on how many calories are in something, we're failing to look at all the other factors that make up that product. Something with zero calories might include harmful chemicals or hidden substances that are bad for us. Something with a ton of calories might be avoided even though it has many vitamins and necessary fiber.

Calories should still be considered, as the more calories you take in, the more you have to burn through exercise. They always shouldn't be a basis for what foods you decide to eat. If you focus too much on calories, you'll end up losing sight of other important issues.

Remember that weight loss isn't about numbers. What's on the scale or the nutrition package is essential in making specific measurements, but they shouldn't be the definitive goals you're creating on your weight-loss journey.

Affirmations

Practicing affirmations is a vital mindset strategy in weight loss. An affirmation is a type of positive reinforcement that helps in combating negative thoughts. Instead of telling yourself you're "no good" because you didn't follow through with a small goal, you should give yourself an affirmation such as "I am capable of continuing" to remind yourself of how powerful you are. Below is a list of positive affirmations you should use to combat negative thoughts and improve overall encouragement:

- I can do this. I am capable of losing weight, and I can reach my goals.

- I am exercising every day and eating healthy as often as possible. I am doing what I should be doing to achieve my goals.

- If I can start my journey, I can finish it.

- I do not need processed foods to feel happy. I can feel the same joy from cooking a healthy meal.

- I have exercised before and can do it again. It is hard to start, but I know that I have what it takes to finish my exercise routine once I do.

- I am healing myself. I have been through challenging times and deserve to feel happy.

- I am loved and am full of love.

- I am losing weight to be healthy.

- I am beautiful no matter what size. Skipping one day at the gym does not mean that I am not beautiful.

- I am eating healthy food full of nourishment. I can feel the positive change in my body, and I know that I only have more to look forward to.

You control the crucial elements that make self-hypnosis work for you. These elements, which might be motivation, belief, and expectation, are the equal components that give you joy or fulfillment for any aim you choose. Let us look at each element and how you may use it to carry out your hypnosis.

Motivation

Motivation is the electricity for your choice of what you want. Wanting is a feeling that you may control. You have managed your preference or looking through limiting it or denying it in most of your lifestyles. You may be superb at handling your goals and wanting in some regions and susceptible or unpracticed in others.

Since that is a "diet" book, you could have already organized yourself to listen that this "diet" will be just like the others that have informed you what you must deny yourself or limit. I.e., the alternative diets have instructed you what no longer to need, and the emphasis may also have been about "no longer trying" a few foods that you have grown to love. Welcome to a fresh way of treating yourself; we can inspire you to get even higher at "looking." We did not cover denial in this guide.

Your motivation is a crucial factor, and one of the fundamental substances. We want you to focus your strength of looking not closer to food, however closer to the incentive that genuinely tells your mind-body what you want it to create: best weight. We inspire you to get in reality desirable at wanting your perfect weight. Here is an example. Let's say you are in a swimming pool, and abruptly you breathe in a mouthful of water.

Time Is on Your Side

You do now not need to worry about how long any patterns or packages have been running on your unconscious or thoughts-frame. They can exchange the instant you discover what needs correction or realignment, as properly as while you make the deliberate choice to alternate them. We would like you to know how your thoughts-frame is familiar with time. You are aware of the linear and mechanical dimension of time in days, hours, minutes, and seconds—what we call "clock time."

That is the way your conscious mind understands the dimension of time. Your unconscious, your mind-frame, handiest understands "now time," where one minute can appear like ten, or ten minutes can seem like one, or the entire thing is happening in the "now." In your sleep, you could revel in a dream occurring inside the region you lived as a child, but with people who went to your high school, human beings you may see at tomorrow's scheduled meeting, and the person who took your order for lunch that day.

All this could arise at the identical time to your dream because your unconscious perceives all time as "now." During your trance work, you may listen to Dr. G. point out that your unconscious can use the hypnotic pointers along with pics and thoughts of destiny as if they have already occurred. Since all time is "now time" to your subconscious, you can adjust, replace, or create the thoughts and programs that you want to "run" within you right "now."

Changed Forever

Roger Bannister, a British athlete, is an excellent example of a person selected to trust himself. Until 1954, when he broke the document time for going for walks the mile in less than four minutes, the arena believed that it's not possible. Yet within three hundred and sixty-five days of his achievement, thirty-seven other runners around the sector additionally ran the mile in less than four minutes.

When your ideas about something alternate, they do now not revert to old ideals that no longer maintain genuinely. As you make adjustments, adjustments, and realignments for your dreams, they're for all time changed. New beliefs are contagious and unfold rapidly.

Check-in with yourself. Tell yourself that your past enjoyment with a weight-reduction plan and weight loss isn't always a predictor of your achievement. Expect your success by using your motivation, beliefs, and expectations. You will see what you accept as real.

Is It All in Your Mind?

Now you'll be thinking maybe the ideas you are studying about ideals and self-hypnosis are "all on your mind." That is a truthful question. It changed into the normal notion that hypnosis became a psychological revel that most effectively involved the mind.

However, studies show that it involves each of the body and mind. A look at the report inside the American Journal of Psychiatry in 2000 used PET brain scans to look at the regions of the mind activated by shade and gray sunglasses.

They found that after the proven result of hypnotized topics, the gray color had changed into the shade, the elements of the mind that method color got activated, and the gray-color processing areas were not.

Research in Neuro-Image in 2004 used useful MRI mind scanning to look at the parts of the mind activated by using ache. Subjects have been given hypnotic pointers to revel in pain. The researchers located that hypnotically precipitated ache and physically produced ache triggered the same components of the brain.

What these studies tell us is, "Yes, it's far in your mind ... and your body." Your body responds to ideas, thoughts, expectations, and hypnotic hints as real, totally, and physically.

For the foremost part, once we are talking about losing weight and ensuring that we will get our health within the right order that we might like, we are getting to focus on exercise and, therefore, the diet. Both of those are important. One goes to make sure that we are ready to reduce and keep our hearts as healthy as possible within the process and is understood to repel tons of the various diseases out there. But the opposite one will help to scale back weight and make sure the body is getting the nutrients it needs.

Slow Down and Chew

We have to start out slowing down when it's time to eat our meals. We'd like to offer the brain a while to process what you're eating and understand once you have had enough to eat. Once you chew the food all the way through, it's getting to force you to hamper in your eating, and it's getting to be associated back with a decreased amount of food that you simply absorb. It can cause you to feel full faster, and you'll combat smaller portion sizes.

How fast you're ready to finish your meals also can have an enormous effect on your current weight. One review done on 23 observational studies found that the people who ate their meals tons faster were more likely to realize weight than the slower eaters. And fast eaters in these studies were also those who are more likely to be obese.

This is a simple thing to repair. You'll set a timer and not allow yourself to eat faster than that at any time. You'll also make it's found out so that you count what percentage times that you chew each bite, then take a drink of water in between. This is often getting to be a simple thanks for assisting you in hampering and can make it easier to eat less at the meal.

Go With Smaller Plates

You will find that the standard food plate may be a lot bigger than it won't be. This is often a trend that's getting to contribute to weight gain because employing a smaller plate can help you eat less as your portions are getting to look tons larger than they are. This is often an honest thanks to making sure that you're getting to trick your mind about what proportion it eats.

On the opposite hand, once you work with a plate that's tons bigger, it's getting to make a serving, a bigger one, look smaller.

You'll be more likely to feature on more food and eat quite you ought to. This suggests that you simply can use this to your advantage. If you're getting to eat tons of healthy foods, accompany the larger plate, so you're taking on bigger portions of it and obtain more of those great things. But if you're getting to eat foods that aren't as healthy, then plow ahead and accompany the smaller plates.

Add within the Protein

Protein goes to possess some powerful effects on appetite. It's ready to help us increase our feelings of fullness, scale back your hunger, and make it easier to eat fewer calories. This might be because protein affects several hormones that play a hunger and fullness task, including the ghrelin hormone.

There is one study that found once we increase our protein intake from 15 percent to 30 percent of our calories, it made it easier for participants to require 441 fewer calories per day then lose 11 pounds over 12 weeks on average, and this was all without intentionally restricting any of the opposite foods that the participants were eating. A good thanks to using this is often together with your meals. If you're eating a breakfast that's filled with grains, for instance, then switching to a meal that's higher in protein could also be an honest place to start. One study found that obese and overweight women who had eggs as a part of their breakfast were ready to eat fewer calories at lunch than those at breakfast based more on grains.

Eat the Fiber

Eating foods rich in fiber is different for us to form sure that we increase our satiety, which helps us feel fuller for an extended period of your time. Studies also show us that one sort of fiber, which is understood as viscous fiber, goes to help when it involves weight loss. This one is so good because it's ready to increase the quantity of fullness that we've, and it's ready to reduce the foods that we intake.

Drink Water Often

We even have to form sure that we are drinking enough water daily because this may help us refill our stomachs so that we eat less and reduce within the process. This is often getting to happen even more once we confirm to drink before a meal. One study in adults found that drinking about 17 ounces of water about half an hour before a meal would help to scale back the quantity of hunger that was felt and help reduce what percentage calories the individual was getting to absorb.

During this study, those who took the time to drink more water before their meals were ready to lose 44 percent more weight over three months than those who didn't have the water before their meals. If you're prepared to replace a number of the regular drinks that you wish to have, which are loaded with calories, like juice or soda, with water, the load loss that you only are experiencing may be going to be even higher.

Keep the Portions Small

In addition to those bigger plates that we were talking about before, you'll find that portion sizes have seen a rise over the past few decades, especially once we leave to eat. These larger portions encourage people to eat more and maybe linked back to an increase in weight and obesity overall.

One study in adults found that when the appetizer with the dinner was doubled, it had been ready to increase the number of calories taken in by 30 percent. You'll find that serving yourself just a touch bit less might be enough to assist you to eat fewer calories, and if it impossible that you simply would even notice the difference.

Don't Eat Neat the TV

Paying more attention to what you're eating could assist you to require fewer calories overall. Those that eat while they're on the pc or watching a show could easily lose track of the quantity they're eating. This is often getting to cause them to overeat also. One review of 24 studies found that those that were distracted once they were eating their meals would consume about 10 percent more during that sitting than those that paid attention.

Besides, being absent-minded when it came to the meal would significantly influence what proportion you took in later within the day. Those that were more distracted during a meal would eat 25 percent more calories at later meals than those that paid more attention. If you're within the habit of consuming meals while watching TV or using some quiet device, then it's likely you're eating more without noticing. These are calories that will add up and may have an enormous impact on your weight over time.

Try to Avoid Stress and Sleep More

Now, if you're a parent, you almost certainly read the thing above and began laughing. Sleeping well and avoiding all of the strain can seem almost impossible once you are a parent, and you've got a bunch of things to stay track of for your children. And if your children aren't sleeping through the night yet, getting that sleep that you simply need could seem almost impossible also. This is often also why tons of oldsters are getting to gain weight when taking care of their children, and it's a real example of why we'd like to pay a touch more attention to our sleeping styles to make sure that we get enough.

Cut Out the Sugary Drinks

Added sugar goes to be one of the worst ingredients that we are ready to increase our diets today. Numerous studies mention how sugary beverages, like soda, are increasing the danger that we've of the many different diseases. It's very easy to consume more calories from these drinks because the calories from a liquid aren't getting to affect our levels of fullness within the same way that a solid food can

These are just a couple of the items that we are ready to neutralize to scale back the quantity that we are eating daily. Once we are ready to make sure that we are just taking within the great things and reducing the amount of the bad stuff that we are consuming, we are getting to see some big changes in our overall health in no time in the least.

These are all simple tasks that you are ready to try and aren't meant to be difficult or too hard to follow. But once we make a couple of small changes, maybe just trying out one or two of those at a time and slowly build-up, we'll find that it's easier than ever to travel through and lose the load that we would like, regardless of what quite a diet plan we are on within the first place.

CHAPTER 22:

Self-hypnosis for extreme weight loss

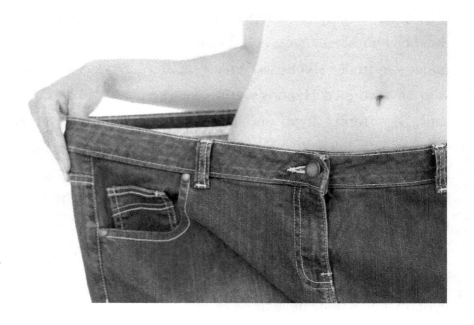

One might ask, "How does hypnosis work?" the solution to the present question isn't definite. The mind has been an enormous puzzle among scientists, and a particular psychological state called Hypnosis may also be a puzzle. The only things that can be said about Hypnosis are the very things that happen in the hypnotic state. These are the behavioral changes and brain activities that a subject undergoes under Hypnosis. What remains a mystery for those who have studied Hypnosis 200 years ago can still be safely said. The term "hypnosis" can be best described as an interaction between two people. If one of the people is trying to influence other people's perceptions, feelings, thinking, and behavior, then the former is called "hypnotist" and the latter the "subject." In this interaction, the hypnotist will ask the subject to concentrate on ideas and images that may evoke the intended responses. The verbal communications that the hypnotist uses to achieve these responses are named "hypnotic suggestions." If a person practiced the hypnotic procedures independently without a hypnotist's help, that activity is called "self-hypnosis."

How Self-Hypnosis Works

Performing self-spellbinding is as basic as having the option to move into a perspective you are in when you are dreaming and resting. The conscious mind in this state is relaxed, and your thoughts can flow freely to and from the subconscious.

Doing this can assist us with a wide range of things. Not exclusively will it assist us with accelerating our weight reduction. However, it can help with sorrow, mending wounds, expanding confidence, assembling a superior body, recuperating inner wounds, relieving disorders, and lots more.

The process is very easy to perform; to begin, locate a decent, calm spot to plunk down, don't rest since you could nod off, and we don't need that to occur. Self-spellbinding for weight reduction can be unwinding and can make us nod off on the off chance that we are not cautious. We will likely have the option to speak with our inner mind. If we are dozing, at that point, this won't occur.

So, when you are plunking down in a suitable position, you can be perched on a seat if this feels the most suitable or on the floor; the best position is one where you are leaning against a divider with your legs loosened up before you.

This position permits you to keep your back straight and feel the vitality stream from your toes to your head; sitting on a seat will also help. In any case, the progression of vitality will be, to some degree, limited due to the bowed knees.

After you are in your agreeable position, loosen up your appendages' entirety and take three full breaths. This causes us to unwind and prepare for our excursion into ourselves.

Next, start by taking a gander at your toes and envision they are loose. Imagine you can see vitality moving upwards from your toes toward your legs.

How to Change Your Thoughts

In the relaxed, attentive state of self-hypnosis, you can be more aware of what are usually "automatic" thoughts. One approach is to use one session to notice and remember the automatic ideas that come up around a particular issue and then write down the thoughts and counter-thoughts you would like to replace them with.

For example, if one of your automatic thoughts was "I never succeed at anything," a counter-thought might be, "I succeed at things often. When I do, I pay attention to them and congratulate myself."

Then, in a second session, you can practice saying the pair of thoughts and gradually shifting the weight of credibility and commitment to the counter-thought.

How to Change Your Feelings

Changing emotions is very feasible with self-hypnosis. A straightforward technique is to connect with the feeling, give it a name (such as "anxiety"), and then notice how it feels in your body.

Imagine what color it would be if it had a color, what texture it would have if it had a texture, what sound it might make. Then imagine that color, texture, or sound changing to one that is more pleasant. Another emotional technique is to imagine your negative feeling on the one hand and a positive feeling you want to replace it with on the other hand. Focus attention on them alternately, gradually bring them together and allow the positive attitude to be dominant as you close your hands together.

How to Change Your Behavior

In self-hypnosis, you can also visualize your future behavior as different from what you currently do in a particular set of circumstances. This mental pre-rehearsal or "future pacing" helps to prepare your mind to behave in that way in real life.

You can also motivate yourself by picturing the positive consequences of changing and comparing them with the negative effects of staying the same.

How to Achieve Your Dreams

If you're clear in your mind about your dreams, you'll have some idea about the thoughts, feelings, and behaviors that belong to someone who's fulfilled those dreams. When you use self-hypnosis to move closer to being that kind of person, your dreams come closer to your grasp.

Emotional Side of Weight Loss and Why It's So Important

Calories in ought to be less than calories out - this is frequently affirmed to be the exact and successful equation of weight reduction. The issue is that the technique doesn't work for some individuals. A solitary explanation exists for that reality - this recipe doesn't factor in the passionate parts of getting in shape.

For some individuals, shedding pounds is a major battle. It incorporates longings, passionate eating, and addictions to specific nourishments. These parts make it inconceivably hard to adequately present change and keep up a person's degree of joy and fulfillment.

Is it true that you are battling with your weight reduction goals? You aren't the only one! A few elements could add to your disappointment, and disregarding the enthusiastic parts of weight addition and misfortune could likewise cause your issues.

The Most Powerful Emotional Components

Several emotional responses could interfere with losing weight and maintenance efforts. The most important ones include:

Anxiety and nervousness: for a few people, these feelings cause enthusiastic eating. When feeling apprehensive, these people need an outlet and a wellspring of solace. Food is much of the time in this outlet. Food "perks up" these people and empowers them to keep working while at the same time holding the adverse feelings within proper limits. Exercise phobia: a passionate component that is regularly thought little of. Numerous individuals accept that activity is unimaginably unpleasant. Some stress over getting to the rec center because of their current weight. They lack motivation, never enjoyed sports, and believe that the situation isn't going to be much different this time. Body image: how do you perceive yourself? The lack of confidence and love for yourself could prevent you from getting to that ideal weight. You may think that you simply don't deserve change or aren't ok to possess a healthy and fit body. This is why you're probably sabotaging your weight loss efforts.

Previously mentioned are not many of the normal intense subject matters remaining inside the fruitful weight reduction method. For certain individuals, it could be much increasingly convoluted. An awful connection with food, compulsion, and reliance is a significantly increasingly genuine mental issue that makes weight reduction unimaginable.

Then Why Do People Fear Hypnosis?

Something that causes individuals to delay utilizing a trance inducer or to utilize self-mesmerizing is that they imagine that entrancing is risky. Indeed, in all cases, the response to this inquiry is that mesmerizing isn't risky. Part of what people seek once they are looking to use a hypnotist is to seek someone who will make them do something they cannot do or don't want.

Furthermore, this idea that they could have this sort of relationship with someone else likewise frightens them. The trance inducer can't transform you into a reluctant member in anything! The trance inducer can just help you with what you're willing and prepared to achieve.

Working with a hypnotist will help you see, feel, and act fully congruent with what you want to accomplish. There's no danger in seeking the assistance of a hypnotist or using self-hypnosis techniques to help you briefly or future goals.

The Key to Making Self-Hypnosis Work

Self-hypnosis has been employed by an excellent many of us to make real, measurable changes in themselves and their lives. Immense quantities of individuals have used the office of self-spellbinding to dispense with fears, control torment, treat physical and mental manifestations, as well as utilizing it to prevail in their objectives.

Notwithstanding, numerous others have accomplished nothing advantageous from its utilization even though specialists state that everybody is hypnotizable! All in all, the inquiry remains - Why doesn't it generally work?

Many people fail to achieve any measurable results from self-hypnosis because they're not using it correctly!

The initial step you should take when considering utilizing self-entrancing is to comprehend what you might want. Despite the fact that this may sound rudimentary and a bit of deigning, truly think about it. Do you know correctly, directly down to the last detail, what you might want to acknowledge from your self-spellbinding project? Or, do you listen to a generic self-hypnosis session and hope for the best?

For example, taking note of a self-hypnosis recording for more confidence could also be an honest goal, but how does one quantify confidence? Do you want to be confident around people or potential mates? It is sheltered to state that you are attempting to recognize more trust in your movement or work-life? Is it actually that you need to be progressively sure about your capacities, and in this way, it is your confidence that you wish to construct?

For self-hypnosis, like all other self-improvement techniques, to be effective, you want to use it with a goal in mind! Your objective, to be utilized with self-mesmerizing, must be exact.

Take a stab at recording a rundown of things you might want to accomplish and afterward organize them. Take your most fundamental want and switch it into an objective. Might you be able to record it? Kindly do it now!

Weight Loss Self Hypnosis

In a supersized world, individuals have numerous chances to eat and drink WAY excessively, yet what's behind corpulence usually is more than longing for a huge request of fries. In America, a genuine eating regimen industry has developed around obesity.

It powers overweight individuals to follow through on a significant expense in vogue diets, pills, or costly and high-hazard medical procedures. By doing away with starches or fat, taking pills or infusions, sprinkling gems on your food, falling back on careful medication, or drinking naturally occurring diet elixirs, numerous health food nuts briefly lose pounds don't lose the outlook which contributes to weight gain.

The outcome is that after such difficult work and conceivably burning through a huge number of dollars, most calorie counters recover their weight and feel significantly progressively disheartened. Weight loss hypnosis can help you change how you feel and control your bad dieting habits.

Why Self-Hypnosis Is A Great Weight Loss Approach

As a whole, we have harmful convictions that impact how we act and think and our practices. A portion of these particular convictions and examples of reasoning to a great extent decide your weight. These could incorporate your disposition toward food and good dieting.

When you make a decent attempt to lose weight, but you are not losing a lot, debilitation makes it simpler to defend droop the cart. You believe, "I'm not losing in any case, so I'd likewise have that hot fudge dessert." Or, "I didn't practice today, so simply overlook it - the week is destroyed."

Weight misfortune mesmerizing trains you to think like flimsy individuals, settle on food choices like these individuals, and eat meager individuals. Despite some reasoning, normally flimsy individuals aren't that way since they generally eat chicken and serve mixed greens with no dressing.

Instead, they recognize what might feel great in their stomachs BEFORE they eat. At that point, they can eat what they need with some restraint and realize when to quit eating depending on how they feel, and see treats as incidental little extravagances, not a day by day need of shoddy nourishment that they later feel sincere and genuinely lousy about eating.

Weight reduction hypnosis advances safe weight reduction. It keeps your mentality positive, in any event, when weight reduction is delayed now and again. While the weight reduction will consistently change a little from week to week, different aftereffects of Hypnosis, for example, developed confidence, unwinding, inspiration, and a quiet perspective, keep on growing. Entrancing changes the association between food and feelings as it re-makes legitimate views toward eating. Since the program doesn't depend on medications and no eating regimens of any sort, Hypnosis is a sound way to deal with weight reduction that can leave you slimmer, progressively loose. With significant changes way, you approach food and your feelings.

Similarly, as with all Hypnosis, the vast majority of individuals can answer recommendations made once they are in a relaxed state. A legitimate trance specialist will assess whether you're the correct contender for weight reduction spellbinding depending on the quality of your craving to change and your readiness to acknowledge preparing and adhere to directions.

CHAPTER 23:

How to use meditation to beat food cravings

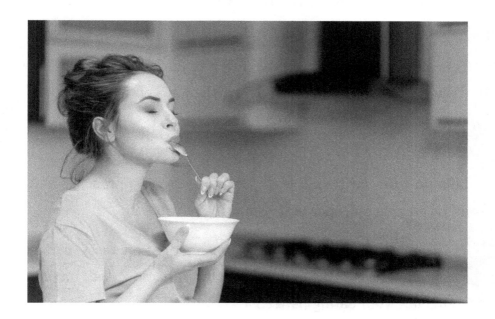

Meditation

Meditation is an activity that helps create a sense of relaxation by linking the body and mind. As a spiritual activity, individuals have been meditating for centuries. Most individuals today use meditation to relieve tension and become more mindful of their emotions.

There are various ways of meditation. A few are focused on the usage of mantras named particular phrases. Others concentrate on the moment of breathing or maintaining consciousness.

Like how the mind and body function, these approaches will help you gain a deeper understanding of yourself.

This enhanced sensitivity allows meditation a valuable technique that might aid in weight reduction and further appreciate your eating patterns.

What's the Link Between Losing Weight and Meditation?

An important method to assist people in losing weight, maybe meditation. What precisely makes meditation in that sense so powerful? It coincides with the unconscious and conscious brain to settle on adjustments we want to add to our actions. These adjustments may involve the regulation of cravings for junk food and the alteration of eating patterns. Having the unconscious mind engaged is crucial since unhealthy, weight-gaining habits such as comfort eating are rooted. Meditation will help you be more mindful about these and overcome them with meditation and substitute them with weight loss practices.

Although meditating provides a more urgent benefit. "The quantities of stress hormones may be decreased explicitly by meditation. Stress hormones like cortisol send our bodies a signal to accumulate energy as fat. When you have a lot of cortisol running into your bloodstream, even though you are making healthier decisions, it would be impossible to lose weight. It sounds difficult, we know; we're all tired, and it seems difficult to undo. But all it takes, a report from Carnegie Mellon University showed, is 25 minutes of mediation three days in a row to relieve tension dramatically.

In reality, volunteers in a 2016 study demonstrated "increased concentration, happiness, calmness, body-mind perception, and brain activation" after only a few short sessions. With everyday practice, self-control may also improve, the study indicates. Researchers discovered that those that enable us to regulate ourselves were the areas of the mind most impacted by meditation. That implies that a few mins of meditation regularly will make it a lot easier to skip that next cookie or skip the ice cream when you feel low.

Knowing the terms regarding weight reduction meditation

Unique strategies and techniques—Meditation, conscientious feeding, and intuitive feeding may help us understand or relearn how to establish a healthier interaction with food and reduce any uncomfortable emotions we could have about nutrition. Losing weight can be a side effect of nurturing this revived friendship, but it is crucial not to develop the primary objective of losing weight. Using so will hinder us such that we cannot feed intuitively or in a deliberate manner.

Instead, reflect on enjoying food, feeding because you need to eat, not because you're exhausted and depressed with work or family problems. You can learn how to respect and value your body and what it can do for you through these lessons.

It will help clarify what the language entails when learning about meditation for losing weight or meditation for nutrition and maintaining a healthier attitude towards food.

Panic or emotional feeding arises when individuals, rather than reacting to their internal signals of hunger, prefer to feed and overeat because of intense emotions or thoughts. Perhaps these thoughts will overshadow our actual sensations of contentment and satiation while we encounter intense emotions, which may contribute to our overeating. Food is used as a calming strategy in these situations, dulling intense feelings temporarily.

However, understanding that this event leads to the perpetuation of a pattern is essential. Experiencing stressful feelings may contribute to overeating, which contributes to remorse or embarrassment, going back to experiencing unpleasant emotions or tension, and not managing or maintaining such situations. Mindful eating is a strategy or process that you may utilize to improve your interaction with food and feeding memories. It requires us to be present and activate our senses, how food tastes, feels, and how it makes our bodies react, most significantly. Mindful eating requires intuitive eating to make us calm down and respond to our inner signals of real desire or signals of pleasure, which will make us limit or even entirely avoid our mental or excessive eating. Even though conscious eating will contribute to weight loss, the objective result or incentive should not lose weight. If our dietary decisions are made based on a certain tangible effect we like, it means that we have already quit actively feeding.

A mind-body, non-diet solution to wellbeing and nutrition is intuitive feeding. To heal our attitude towards food, it opposes the idea of dieting and encourages us to embrace our bodies and respond to our internal bodily signs. Intuitive eating involves conscious eating concepts; however, it also contains a broader generalized concept that extends throughout, pushing the body because it feels nice to walk, often without judgment utilizing diet evidence.

When Exercise and Diet Don't Seem To Be Effective, How Will Meditation Help?

Stress is the leading cause of unnecessary weight gain or the failure to lose weight successfully in certain situations. But, if you've been eating correctly and exercising but are continually anxious, you may not be tackling the core reason for weight gain.

Stress again activates hormones that accumulate excess fat, just what we don't like! This can also fuel a tension cycle: when you're anxious, you can't lose weight, which leaves you frustrated over not reaching your goal. Being caught in a simple process, but you can crack it, and meditation can assist.

It would be best to consider what triggers stress in your life to cope with tension or remove it properly.

Few stressors are easy to spot, but others may be more elusive. I consider utilizing Well Be to grasp better, map, and deal with tension.

The WellBe is a device that acts much like a sensor of movement, but now it is the first of its sort to concentrate on mental health. It also shows you how and what behaviors in your life induce emotional tension and will also support you come up with better coping strategies that will help you lose weight.

How to Meditate

There are lots of ways of meditating.

Most forms of meditation have the following four points in common:

- A quiet place. Can you decide where to meditate — your preferred chair? During a walk? It depends on you.

- A certain relaxed pose, such as lying, sitting, standing, or moving.

- A focus of awareness. You may concentrate on a phrase or expression, your breathing, or anything else.

- A transparent mind. Getting other thoughts when you meditate is natural. Try not to be drawn in those feelings so much. Continue to put your focus back to your voice, word, or something else you're focused on.

- Pick the location you want to try, the time, and the process. To understand the fundamentals, you may even take a lesson.

Instantly, meditation won't help you lose weight.

But it will have lifelong impacts on not just your weight but also your thinking processes with a little practice.

Loss of Sustainable Weight

You can recognize all of these things through mindfulness meditation without judgment.

Meditation is related to several advantages. In terms of weight reduction, mindfulness meditation appears to be the most beneficial. A 2017 study of current research showed that mindfulness meditation was a successful tool for weight reduction and improving eating behaviors.

Meditation for Mindfulness means paying careful attention to:

- Where you are

- Whatever you do,

- The way you feel at the current moment.

- Learn to handle your acts and emotions as they are, nothing more. Take inventory of what:

- You experience and do but strive not to categorize something as fair or poor. Through daily practice, everything gets simpler.

Exercising mindfulness meditation may contribute to long-term effects, too. As per the 2017 study, many who cultivate mindfulness are more likely to hold the weight off relative to other dieters.

Methods of meditation

Conscious Meditation.

It's easy to get caught up in a loop of spinning thoughts — starting to think about a laundry list of activities to do, ruminating about past events, or potentially future situations — and practicing mindfulness may help. Yet what exactly is attention? It can be described as a mental state that requires being fully engaged on "the now" so that, without judgment, you can understand and acknowledge your thoughts, feelings, and sensations.

Mindfulness meditation

Mindfulness meditation is the method of having your thoughts fully present. Knowledge involves being mindful of where we are and what we do and not being too sensitive to what is happening around us.

One can do reflective meditation anywhere. Some people like to sit in a quiet spot, close their eyes, and focus on their respiration. But at every stage of the day, even when driving to work or doing chores, you can choose to be conscious.

You track your thoughts and feelings while practicing mindfulness meditation but let them move without judgment.

Directed Meditation.

Directed meditation, often also referred to as guided imagery or visualization, is a meditation technique in which you create mental images or scenarios that you find calming.

Guided meditation is among the most common methods of meditation employed every day by millions of people. In this post, we'll explore guided meditation and how to do it.

In the purest form, guided meditation is a type of meditation where the individual is guided on every step of his daily practice. Someone directs you right from the first level of sitting in a meditative pose to the final phase of completing the meditation. What occurs is that during meditation, a teacher or mentor provides step-by-step guidance about what to do. It is an ancient method of conveying directions for meditation to pupils. In older times, this technique has been used to teach meditation in a group. Nowadays, thanks to technological development, we no longer need a guru's physical presence to lead us in meditation. We can listen to a master's direct guidance using pre-recorded CDs or DVDs and conduct our meditation practice. In the absence of any meditation master professional CDs / DVDs, you can record guided meditation instructions from a book in your voice and then play them afterward.

Vipassana Meditation.

Vipassana meditation is an ancient form of Indian meditation, which means seeing things as they are. More than 2,500 years ago, it was taught in India. The conscious meditation movement has origins in this practice in the United States.

The purpose of meditation with vipassana is self-transformation through the examination of oneself. This is accomplished to create a deep connection between mind and body by careful attention to the body's sensations. The sustained interconnectedness leads to a happy account, filled with love and compassion.

Vipassana is usually taught during a 10-day course in this tradition. People are expected to follow a set of rules all the time and abstain from all intoxicants, telling lies, cheating, sexual activity, and killing any animals.

Loving Meditation on Compassion (Metta Meditation).

Metta meditation, also called meditation on loving-kindness, is the practice of guiding good wishes towards others.

Those who practice reciting similar words and phrases will elicit warm-hearted sentiments. This is also commonly found in meditation on mindfulness and vipassana.

It's usually done in a pleasant, relaxed position while sitting. After a few deep breathes, you slowly and steadily repeat the following words. "Just let me be happy. May I be fine. Let me be free. May I be calm and at ease". After a period of guiding this loving-kindness to yourself, you may begin to imagine a family member or friend who has supported you and repeat the mantra, this time replacing " I " with" you." As you continue the meditation, you may bring to mind other members of your family, friends, neighbors or people in your life. Practitioners are often encouraged to consider individuals who are having trouble with them.

Meditation Yoga.

The yoga practice has its roots in ancient India. There are various yoga classes and styles, but all include performing a series of postures and guided breathing exercises designed to encourage flexibility and relax the mind.

The poses require balance and attention, and practitioners are encouraged to concentrate less on distractions and remain more at the moment.

Which meditation style you choose to try depends on several factors. When you have a health problem and are new to yoga, tell your doctor what method would be right for you

CHAPTER 24:

What is mindful eating

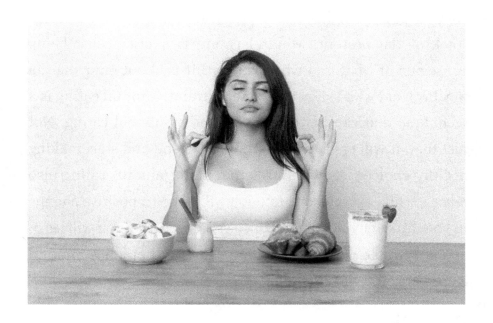

Mindfulness is a simple concept that states that you must be aware of and present in the moment. Often, our thoughts tend to wander, and we might lose track of the present moment. Maybe you are preoccupied with something that happened or are wondering about something that might occur. When you do this, you tend to lose track of the present. Mindful eating is a practice of being conscious of what and when you eat. It is about enjoying the meal you eat while showing some restraint. Mindful eating is a technique that can help you overcome emotional eating. Not just that, it will teach you to enjoy your food and start making healthy choices. As with any other skill, mindful eating also takes a while to inculcate, but you will notice a positive change in your attitude toward food once you do. In this, you will learn about a couple of simple tips you can use to practice mindful eating in your daily life.

Reflection

Before you start eating, take a minute and reflect upon how and what you are feeling. Are you experiencing hunger? Are you feeling stressed? Are you bored or sad? What are your wants, and what do you need? Try to differentiate between these two concepts. Once you are done reflecting for a moment, you can now choose what you want to eat, if you do want to eat and how you want to eat.

Sit Down

It might save some time if you eat while you are working or while traveling to work. Regardless of what it is, you must ensure that you sit down and eat your meal.

Please don't eat on the go, instead set a couple of minutes aside for your mealtime. You will not be able to appreciate the food you are eating if you are trying to multitask. It can also be quite difficult to keep track of all the food you eat when eating on the go.

No Gadgets

If all your attention is focused on the TV, your laptop, or anything else that comes with a screen, it is unlikely that you will be able to concentrate on the meal that you are eating. When your mind is distracted, you tend to indulge in mindless eating. So, limit your distractions or eliminate them if you want to practice mindful eating.

Portion your Food

Don't eat straight out of a container, a bag, or a box. When you do this, it becomes rather difficult to keep track of the portions you eat, and you might overindulge without even being aware of it. Not just that, you will never learn to appreciate the food you are eating if you keep doing this.

Small Plates

We are all visual beings. So, if you see less, your urge to eat will also decrease. It is a good idea to start using small plates when you are eating.

You can always go back for a second helping, but this is a simple way to regulate the quantity of food you keep wolfing down.

Be Grateful

Before you dig into your food, take a moment, and be grateful for all the labor and effort that went into providing the meal you are about to eat.

Acknowledge that you are lucky to have the meal you do, which will help create a positive relationship with food.

Chewing

It is advised that you must chew each bite of food at least thirty times before swallowing it. It might sound tedious but make it a point to chew your food at least ten times before you swallow.

Take this time to appreciate the flavors, textures, and taste of the food you are eating. Apart from this, when you thoroughly chew the food before swallowing, it helps with better digestion and absorption of food.

Clean Plate

You don't have to eat everything that you serve on your plate. I am not suggesting that you must waste food. If you have overfilled your plate, don't overstuff yourself. You must eat only what your body needs and not more than that. So, start with small portions and ask for more helpings. Overstuffing yourself will not do you any good, and it is equivalent to mindless eating.

Prevent Overeating

It is important to have well-balanced meals daily. You shouldn't skip any meals, but it doesn't mean that you should overeat. Eat only when you feel hungry and don't eat otherwise. Here are a couple of simple things you can do to avoid overeating. Learn to eat slowly. It isn't a new concept, but not many of us follow it. We are always in a rush these days. Take a moment and slow down. Take a sip of water after every couple of bites and chew your food thoroughly before you gulp it down. Don't just mindlessly eat and learn to enjoy the food you eat. Concentrate on the different textures, tastes, and flavors of the food you eat. Learn to savor every bite you eat and make it an enjoyable experience. Make your first-bit count and let it satisfy your taste buds. Now is the time to let your inner gourmet chef out! Use a smaller plate while you eat, and you can easily control your portions. Stay away from foods that are rich in calories and wouldn't satiate your hunger. Fill yourself up with foods that can satisfy your appetite and make you feel full for longer. If you have a big bowl of salad, you will feel fuller than you would if you have a small bag of chips. The calorie intake might be the same for both these things, but the hunger you will feel afterward differs.

The idea is to fill yourself up with healthy foods before you think about junk food. While you eat, make sure that you turn off all electronic gadgets. You tend to lose track of the food you eat while you watch TV.

Practicing Mindfulness

Mindfulness meditations help you put some space between yourself and how you react whenever you face any situation. The following practices will guide you to tune into mindful meditation daily:

Set aside some time - All you need is to set aside some time from your busy schedule to engage in meditations. Getting off other activities is the most crucial requirement for effective mindful mediation. Observe your present moment as it is - The goal of mindfulness is to give close consideration to what you are encountering at the immediate moment without judging it. It is not about quieting your mind or attempting to achieve some state of long-lasting calm.

Focus on the sensations, thoughts, and imaginations of your mind at that present moment.

Let your judgments pass - In case you notice any thoughts during your practices, you shouldn't suppress them. Instead, take a mental note of them and let them pass.

Return to the present moment - Once your judgments have passed, focus back your mind to the present, making observations of the current as it is. Mindfulness is about returning your thoughts to the present, sometimes several, during your entire practice.

Your mind tends to carry off easily by the myriads of thoughts crossing it. You must refocus your mind on the present thought.

Don't judge your wandering - You shouldn't be hard on yourself every time your mind wanders off during the practice. It is common for all humans to have thoughts propping up instinctively, and without any warning, you should, therefore, learn how to recognize when your mind wandered off to bring it back and refocus it on the present gently.

Important Mindfulness Techniques

We can practice mindfulness in different ways.

All of the available methods focus on how you can achieve a state of alertness and relaxation to focus your attention on your thoughts and sensations without judging them. The following are some of the meditation techniques:

Basic mindfulness technique

This technique requires you to sit quietly in the same spot and focus on your breathing. You can also focus on saying a single word that you silently say over and over again. You should allow your thoughts to come in and out without judgment, and each time, you return to your focus on the breath.

Body sensations

You ought to likewise observe little and inconspicuous body sensations, for example, an itch or shivering. Try not to pass judgment on the senses. Instead, permit them to pass. It would help if you observed all emotions occurring in all aspects of your body, from your head to the toe.

Sensory

You should also note the sensory sensations such as the sights, sounds, smells, touches, or taste. Give them names and let them pass without any judgment.

Emotions

You should also let your emotions manifest without suppressing or judging them. You should name your feelings in a steady and relaxed way, such as "joy, anger, happiness."

Cravings and urges

You should let your cravings for addictive substances or behaviors to be present. Allow them to pass without judgment. Take a conscious mental note of how your body feels when the specific cravings enter.

How to Incorporate Mindfulness into Your Daily Life?

Mindfulness can be practiced anywhere and at any time of the day. No law limits mindfulness to sitting on a cushion.

You can incorporate the essential techniques of mindfulness into your everyday activities and tasks. Such events provide a lot of opportunities for you to carry out your mindfulness practice. You can cultivate mindfulness in your daily routine through some of the following practices:

While Washing Dishes

When you are busy doing the dishes, you hardly get any distractions from everyone else. The fact that you get little distractions when doing the dishes offers you an excellent opportunity to try some mindfulness.

As you clean your dishes and kitchen, you should train your mind to focus on the physical activity, making a note of the warm water on your hand, the sound of the clanking utensils, and the sound of the running water. All these activities and their accompanying sensations will help your mind focus on the present.

Brushing Your Teeth

You brush your teeth daily, sometimes more than twice each day. This could offer you an excellent opportunity to practice mindfulness meditation. Take note of the brush in your hand, the feet on the ground, and how your arm moves up and down as you undertake your brushing.

Driving

It is relatively easy to let your mind wander off when you are driving, but you should use your mindfulness power to anchor your thoughts to the present, focusing on the inside of your car. You can start by turning off your car radio or putting on some cool, soothing music. Then gently bring back your mind to the present, paying attention to where you are and what you are experiencing.

Exercising

You can practice mindfulness while atop your treadmill. Just focus on your breathing and where your feet are in space as you work on your treadmill. Pay close attention to the way you take in and out your breath. Notice how the pattern your legs create as your feet hit the mill or the ground.

CHAPTER 25:

Benefits of Intuitive Eating

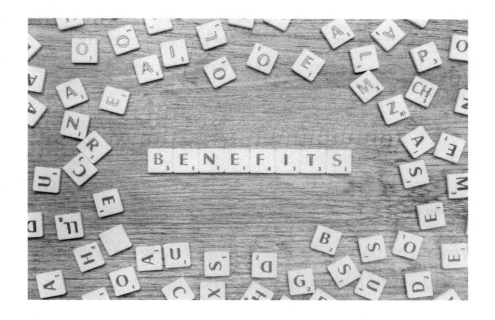

Intuitive eating isn't intended for weight reduction. Sadly, there might be dietitians, mentors, and different experts that sell intuitive eating as a diet, which runs counter to the thought altogether. The objective of intuitive eating is improving your association with food. This incorporates building more beneficial food practices and making an effort not to control the scale. That being stated, pretty much everyone experiencing the way toward figuring out how to be an intuitive eater needs to get thinner—else, they'd as of now be intuitive eaters!

Intuitive eating enables your body to break the diet cycle and sink into its regular set point weight territory. This might be lower, higher, or a similar weight you are at present.

How Intuitive Eating Plays a Role in Healthy Living and Shopping Lifestyle:

Intuitive eating guides our lives inside and out. It creates such a lot of opportunity and straightforwardness by not stressing over what I will eat or when I will eat it. I stream with what my body guides me to eat, and when it guides me to it eat-and with that, it creates opportunity inside my relationship in my body and how I feel about myself. I am more advantageous and more adjusted than I have ever been in my body, and I can say that I love my body and this vessel that I am carrying on with this life in.

This move-in my association with my body, food, and general surroundings is an immediate consequence of my otherworldly voyage.

The most significant thing is not to stress over the 'right' or 'wrong' choice, and instead to distinguish how you are feeling and where in your body you think it is the goal you aren't eating to keep away from concealing feelings. That way, you're eating decisions are simpler to make since they aren't enveloped with your passing feelings.

There is such a lot of opportunity and facilitate that shows up when you interface with and pursue your instinct. Shopping for food turns out to be, to a lesser degree, a task or a problem and increasingly an action of happiness and articulation. To have the option to purchase what looks, sounds, and scents great (offers to the faculties) and believe my instinct as far as what I will cook and create each day/week. It also makes the creation procedure progressively fun since you don't feel adhered to pursuing a formula or dinner plan. Once more, there is an opportunity. Shopping for food is only an expansion of that and part of the creation procedure (where motivation comes in).

Indeed, there might, in any case, be times when you don't feel like shopping for food or preparing; however, in those minutes, you aren't hung up on it. The dread of settling on a wrong choice or eating inappropriate food vanishes. Intuitive eating isn't about control and dread; it is about the stream and following what feels better (from a space of instinct, not damage or self-hurt).You are beginning the adventure of understanding what foods reverberate with your body and what doesn't-interfaces with the act of enthusiastic mindfulness. On the off chance that we shut ourselves off from feeling our feelings, at that point, we are additionally closing down our capacity to feel different sensations. Consider it like this-your body is sending you the flag of what feels better and what doesn't; however, you have unplugged the wire association between the inclination, and you are accepting and being informed of the disposition. Having an essential comprehension of sustenance is a great spot to start teaching oneself and acclimate oneself with specific establishments of pure sciences. From that point, it truly is an act of backing off and carrying your attention to how you feel during and after eating. At whatever point you notice examples of side effects, you should investigate. What musings did you see, how could you feel, what was going on around then? A great deal of our food and eating practices/designs have been adapted and created quite a while prior and requires bringing our cognizance again into that space to develop progressive movements. The most significant piece of this procedure is to curry sympathy with you and practice non-judgment.

The diet culture is a finished square to instinct. It is established in dread, and control-and expels the opportunity to interface with how you feel or what your body wants. The diet culture mirrors the longing to change and control the body instead of helping it and work with it. It is tied in with stifling the body's direction framework (through control), which expels you further away from your instinct and the capacity to interface with your intuition through your body's informing structure. The greatest thing to perceive is that your body is profoundly insightful and realizes what to do-the more that you work with it and backing (and trust it)- the more joyful you will feel. At whatever point we hop onto a pattern, it is imperative to associate with what feels better (and inquire whether this pattern genuinely impacts you or on the off chance that you are merely doing it since others are, and their outcomes entice you). A great spot to ground yourself in what your intuitive direction is, is to ask yourself, "What feels useful for your spirit?"

The Health Benefits of Intuitive Eating

Improvement in Digestion:

- Two of the fundamental precepts of intuitive eating are to:

- Eat just when you're ravenous,

- Eat until you're fulfilled, not stuffed.

- Rehearsing both of these propensities can help improve your assimilation in various manners.

For one, eating just when you're genuinely hungry gives your stomach related framework time to discharge your stomach from your last supper. This may appear no major ordeal, and however, when you continue eating each couple of hours and not enabling your food to process, your framework can undoubtedly move toward becoming exhausted. Your stomach needs to consistently siphon out chemicals and acids to help digest your food, while your liver is ceaselessly being attempted to channel poisons and condensation fat.

Additionally, eating until you're full at each feast can shield your assimilation from running comfortably. You're basically "Backing up" your framework by pouring undigested food over half-processed food, which may make you experience acid reflux, stoppage, or any number of stomach related issues.

Rehearsing body mindfulness, eating just until you're fulfilled, and not eating between suppers except if you're eager gives your stomach related framework a rest with the goal that it's completely prepared to deal with your dinner.

There Is No Room for Stress:

Studies have demonstrated that intuitive eaters not just appreciate a more lovely enthusiastic state than dieters, yet additionally experience enhancements in despair, nervousness, negative self-talk, and general mental prosperity when they change to eating intuitively.

The explanation behind this decrease in pressure may originate from how you get the chance to concentrate more on making the most of your food instead of dissecting it when you eat intuitively. You additionally remove yourself from the outlook of, "I can't have that since I have to get thinner," or "I can't have carbs because I'm fat."

These sorts of responses to food put a heap of weight at the forefront of your thoughts and body, so it's no big surprise you feel better when you let them go!

A Possibility to Aid Weight Loss:

Studies have likewise indicated that intuitive eaters have lower weight records (BMIs) than dieters. One of the significant purposes behind this could be that intuitive eating is anything but difficult to adhere to (not at all like trend diets), which can prompt long haul weight reduction.

When you eat intuitively, you also figure out how to regard a satiety flag that discloses to you when you're fulfilled versus only eating for eating. This outcome in a natural, ideal calorie balance could prompt weight reduction on the off chance you've been overeating by disregarding yearning signs.

Intuitive eating lessens feelings of anxiety can likewise assume a job since a lot of the pressure hormone cortisol can cause fat addition.

High Self-Esteem:

Notwithstanding improving eating examples and nervousness levels, contemplates have additionally demonstrated that rehearsing intuitive eating develops confidence.

For example, members in a single report experienced more acknowledgments of their bodies and less mental pain concerning their bodies. They were additionally ready to relinquish "Unfortunate weight control practices."

By improving your confidence, it's just typical that different parts of your life will improve too. At the point when you're concentrating less on not being "Sufficient" and more on tolerating yourself, you'll generally encounter less nervousness and have an increasingly inspirational point of view. Thus, this can prompt many open doors at work and enhancements in your connections.

A Decent Improvement in Body Awareness:

Monitoring your body and what it's motioning to you is critical with regards to keeping up your wellbeing. On the off chance that you listen intently, your body will offer you inconspicuous hints that something isn't right, enabling you to give it what it needs before it turns into a significant issue.

Take, for instance, indications of supplement inadequacies. Numerous individuals are so separated from their bodies that they don't see hidden signs of a supplement insufficiency, similar to an absence of vitality or shivering in their grasp and feet. When they understand, the inadequacy has turned out to be dangerous to such an extent that they need to go to the specialist to get it dealt with.

Intuitive eating is tied in with connecting with your body's sign of craving and satiety. Be that as it may, you'll begin to be hyper-mindful of different signs your body is emitting when you start focusing on these signs. This will enable you to be in line with what you need consistently, so you can deal with it before it turns into an all-out issue

CHAPTER 26:

Gastric band hypnosis

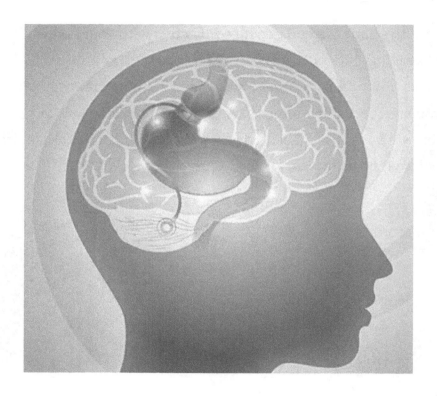

A stomach band is a silicone flexible apparatus utilized in weight reduction in medical procedures. To create a modest pack over the gadget, the band is put around the belly's upper part. This restrains the amount of sustenance that can be put away in the stomach area, making eating enormous amounts hard.

A gastric band will likely constrain the amount of sustenance that an individual can expend physically, making them feel full in the wake of eating next to no to advance weight reduction. It is a final hotel for most people who have this medical procedure after endeavoring for other weight reduction systems. Like any medical procedure, there are perils in fitting a gastric band.

Gastric Band Trance

Gastric band trance can be utilized without the perils that accompany medical procedures to help people get thinner. Numerous trance specialists use a two-dimensional procedure. The first hope to characterize your enthusiastic eating's underlying driver.

Utilizing trance, the specialist can urge you to recall long-overlooked nourishment related encounters that may now influence you subliminally. Before performing gastric band hypnotherapy, tending to and perceiving any unfortunate reasoning, examples concerning sustenance can help.

Next, the trance specialist will play out the treatment of the virtual stomach band. The technique is proposed to recommend that you had an activity to embed a gastric band at a subliminal stage. The objective is to cause your body to respond to this proposition by making you feel quicker as though you had an actual medical procedure.

How it Functions

How gastric band spellbinding works using unwinding a trance specialist techniques will get you a trance condition. Your subliminal is progressively open to proposal in this casual state. Trance inducers are making proposals to your intuitive at this stage. With hypnotherapy of the gastric band, this suggestion is that you have joined a physical band.

The psyche is solid, so your conduct will change as needs be on the off chance that you are subliminal that acknowledges these proposals. More often than not, alongside the virtual gastric band's' fitting,' proposals will be created about trust and conduct to help you focus on this way of life move.

Numerous specialists will likewise encourage strategies for self-mesmerizing so you can improve your activity after the session. It is regularly prescribed to instruct yourself on nourishment and exercise to help physical wellbeing and prosperity.

The Process

Your first subliminal specialist session will likely be a unique counsel to talk about what you would like to get from hypnotherapy. This is an opportunity to talk about any past endeavors at weight reduction, eating rehearses, medical issues, and generally speaking, nourishment frame of mind. This information will furnish the advisor with a clearer idea of what will help and whether to think about some other treatment methods.

The activity itself is expected to imitate the gastric band's medical procedure to help your subliminal think it has happened. Numerous subliminal specialists will incorporate the sounds and scents of a working performance center to make the experience increasingly true. Your specialist will begin by carrying you to a condition of profound unwinding, otherwise called entrancing. You'll be aware of what's happening, and you'll generally be in order.

The specialist will address you through the system once you're sleep-inducing. They will explain bit by bit what is happening in a medical procedure, from being put under a sedative to making the primary entry point, fitting the band itself, and sewing the cut. A working auditorium's sounds and scents will improve the experience to persuade your inner mind that what is said is transpiring.

As expressed before, different proposals to improve self-assurance might be incorporated during the activity. Endless supply of the system, your trance inducer may show you a few strategies for self-spellbinding to help you stay at home on the track.

Some subliminal specialists will approach you to return for follow-up arrangements to screen the virtual band's accomplishment and roll out any improvements. When people also fit the physical band, proceeding with hypnotherapy sessions as a feature of long-term weight management, the board plan might be valuable for a few. This empowers the subliminal specialist to work with you to handle the hidden sustenance and confidence issues.

How am I going to feel afterward?

The general objective of the gastric band is to encourage a more beneficial nourishment association. If your subliminal thinks you have a gastric band fitted, your stomach will believe it's lower. This, thus, makes your mind send messages that, in the wake of devouring less nourishment, you are finished.

Perceiving when you are physically finished can be hard for the individuals who gorge. At times we eat only for taste (or comfort), overlooking whether we are physically hungry or not. In developing smart dieting, figuring out how to perceive the physical vibes of being ravenous and finished is helpful.

In contrast to gastric band medical procedures, there are no physical symptoms in the virtual gastric band. The whole medical procedure may trigger the reflux of queasiness, regurgitating, and corrosive, for a few. Since the gastric band's mesmerizing is not a physical technique, it won't trigger such side effects.

The activity ought to be a charming and loosening up understanding, with most people revealing from entrancing an impression of quiet.

Is it going to work for me?

For the individuals who first attempt hypnotherapy, a well-known issue is - is it getting down to business for me? It is anything but a simple circumstance of yes or no, lamentably; it's mostly up to you. Hypnotherapy empowers people with an assortment of issues. However, it is instrumental in evolving propensities. Hence, helping people make excellent eating practices and shedding pounds is frequently viable. Like some other weight reduction plot, be that as it may, it will include your full commitment.

If you think simultaneously and your specialist, you're bound to get what you need from gastric band hypnotherapy. It is indispensable to be agreeable and to confide in your subliminal specialist. In this manner, it is prescribed that you require significant investment in your district to examine subliminal specialists and discover progressively about them, how they work, and what their aptitudes involve. Before the strategy, you can mastermind to meet them to ensure you are alright with them.

In case you're devoted to changing your way of life, think the methodology, and trust your subliminal specialist, the mesmerizing of the gastric band should work for you.

Using Hypnosis to Control Food Portions

Portion control can assume an amazing job in achieving your objectives for wellbeing and weight. You may, as of now, eat all the right sustenance and practice appropriately. In any case, in case regardless you're conveying overabundance weight, it may be because you're merely expending excessively. Control of segments can make a huge distinction.

Excellent portion control won't just thin you down; it will give you more vitality. Eating the right amount will suggest that your body needs to work more enthusiastically to process superfluous surplus nourishment.

Regarding getting your eating regimen right and shedding surplus fat, the amount is as fundamental as quality. If you have to get thinner, a lot of a decent thing can truly be terrible for you. However, knowing how, when, and the amount to cut so you can truly begin seeing some improvement in accomplishing your weight targets can be troublesome.

Why is Portion control so Hard to Achieve?

Propensity controls our lives substantially more than we understand. We eat because it's an ideal opportunity to eat (even though you had a nibble simply 30 minutes prior).

We're gorging out of good manners, or not having any desire to' squander' what's on our plate, or because we're so used to being full that we've overlooked how to perceive when we've had enough.

Some good judgment things can enable you to control the size of the bit:

- You can eat all the more gradually intentionally. This offers your stomach the chance to enlist its totality in your cerebrum and mood killer your hunger.

- You can begin your supper with soup-it very well may be fulfilling to have a low-calorie soup and enable you to feel cheerful for your fundamental course with a lot of little parts.

- You can utilize the old stunt of the little plate-so you need to eat littler segments truly.

- You can stay away from smorgasbords

Hypnosis is an incredible asset for controlling portions.

In any case, extraordinary as all the exhortation above maybe, despite everything, you have to conquer propensity and impulse, which is the place spellbinding can help. Nourishment is fuel, and the correct quality and amount of fuel are required. Envision attempting to place more fuel when it's full in your vehicle. It's simply not appearing well and good.

Portion control will take you to a profoundly loosened upstate and rapidly train your oblivious personality to intuitively realize when to disregard overabundance sustenance and make your assimilation considerably more agreeable. You will rediscover the joy of being tuned in to the dietary necessities of your own body.

The Power of the Gastric Band

A renowned and dramatic case of hypnotic power to influence our bodies directly is in the emergency treatment of burns. A few doctors have used hypnotic to accelerate and improve the recuperating of extreme injuries and help reduce the excruciating pains for his patients. If somebody is seriously burnt, there will be damage to the tissue, and the body reacts with inflammation. The patients are hypnotized to forestall the soreness. His patients heal quite rapidly and with less scarring.

There are a lot more instances of how the mind can directly and physically influence the body. We realize that chronic stress can cause stomach ulcers, and a psychological shock can turn somebody's hair into a grey color overnight. In any case, I especially like this aspect of hypnotism because it is an archived case of how the mind influences the body positively and medically. It will be somewhat of a miraculous event if the body can get into a hypnotic state that can cause significant physical changes in your body. Hypnotic trance without anyone else has a profound physiological effect. The most immediate effect is that subjects discover it deeply relaxing. Interestingly, the most widely recognized perception that my customers report after I have seen them—regardless of what we have been dealing with—is that their loved ones tell them they look more youthful.

Cybernetic Loop

Your brain and body are in constant correspondence in a cybernetic loop: they continually influence one another. As the mind unwinds in a trance, so too does the body. When the body unwinds, it feels good, and it sends that message to the brain, which thus feels healthier and unwinds much more. This procedure decreases stress and makes more energy accessible to the immune system of the body. It is essential to take note that the remedial effects of hypnotics don't require tricks or amnesia. For example, burns patients realize they have been burnt, so they don't need to deny the glaring evidence of how burnt parts of their bodies are. He practically hypnotizes them and requests that they envision cool, comfortable sensations over the burnt area. That imaginative activity changes their body's response to the burns.

The enzymes that cause inflammation are not released, and accordingly, the burn doesn't advance to a more elevated level of damage, and there is reduced pain during the healing process.

Using hypnotic and imagery, a doctor can get his patients' bodies to do things that are totally outside their conscious control. Willpower won't make these sorts of changes, but the creative mind is more grounded than the will. By using hypnotic and imagery to talk to the conscious mind, we can have a physiological effect in as little as 20 minutes

One and a half days after, the eczema was gone. With hypnotic, we can enormously enhance the effect of the mind. When we fit your hypnotic gastric band, we use the same strategy of hypnotic correspondence to the conscious mind. We communicate to the brain with distinctive imagery. The brain alters your body's responses, changing your physical response to food, so your stomach is constricted, and you feel truly full after only a few.

Visualization Is Easier Than You Think

The hypnotic we use to make your gastric band uses "visualization" and "influence loaded imager." Visualization is the creation of pictures in your mind. We would all be able to do it. It is an interesting part of the reasoning. For instance, think about your front door and ask yourself which side the lock is on. To address that question, you see an image in your mind's eye. It doesn't make a difference at all how reasonable or bright the image is, it is only how your mind works, and you see as much as you have to see. Influence loaded imagery is the psychological term for genuinely significant pictures. In this process, we use pictures in the mind's eye that have emotional significance.

Although hypnotic recommendations are incredible, they are dramatically upgraded by ground-breaking images when communicating directly to the body. For instance, you will be unable to accelerate your heart just by telling it to beat faster. Still, if you envision remaining on a railroad line and seeing a train surging towards you, your heart accelerates pretty quickly. Your body overreacts to clear, meaningful pictures.

It doesn't make a difference whether you are listening intentionally; your conscious mind will hear all it needs to recreate the real band, in a similar way that a clear image of a moving toward train rushing towards your influences your pulse rate. You do not have to hold the pictures of the operational procedures in your conscious mind because you are anesthetized and unconscious during an activity. Notwithstanding what you intentionally recollect, underneath the hypnotic anesthesia, your conscious mind uses this information and imagery to introduce your gastric band in the right spot.

Forms of Gastric Banding Procedures Used in Weight Reduction Hypnotherapy

Sleeve gastrectomy

This operation requires cutting half of a person's stomach, usually the size of a banana, to leave behind space. It will not be reversed once this portion of the stomach is cut away. This can sound like one of the more severe forms of gastric band operation, and it also poses several complications due to its degree of extremity. It does not sound worth it. However, it has been one of the more common procedures used in surgery as a restricting way of suppressing a patient's desire. For those who struggle with obesity, it is beneficial. As per medical experts, it has a reasonable performance rate and relatively few risks. Those who received the surgery suffered a reduction of up to 50% of their overall weight, which is quite a lot for those with obesity.

For others who struggle with compulsive eating problems, including binge eating, it is similarly effective.

A physician will make either a very wide or a pair of minor incisions in the abdomen as you get the surgery performed. It can take up to six weeks to heal from this operation physically.

Vertical banded gastroplasty

This gastric band treatment, commonly known as VBG, includes the same band positioned across the stomach during the sleeve gastrostomy. To shape a tight pouch, the stomach is then fastened above the band, which shrinks the gut in some manner to achieve the same results. Compared to several other forms of weight reduction treatment, the treatment has been recognized as a good one to reduce weight. While it might sound like a less complicated operation relative to a sleeve gastrostomy, it has a higher complication risk. This is why it is found much less prevalent. As of today, this unique gastric band operation is conducted by just 5% of bariatric specialists. Nevertheless, it is renowned for delivering outcomes and can also be used without hypnotherapy problems to achieve comparable effects.

Mixed Surgery (Restrictive and Malabsorptive)

A key feature in certain forms of weight reduction surgery is this method of gastric band operation. It is most generally referred to as a gastric bypass, which is conducted first, preceding all weight reduction procedures. It also contains stomach stapling and makes an intestinal form down your stomach. This is required to guarantee that the patient eats less food in conjunction with malabsorptive surgery, pointed to as a restrictive mixed procedure, ensuring that the body eats less food.

Everything You Need to Understand Regarding Gastric-Band Hypnotic Therapy

You may want to suggest doing the hypnotherapy component if you're unsure if the gastric band procedure is appropriate for you. Hypnotherapy is the ideal solution, as compared to an operation that has several risks, is 100 percent safer and, therefore, far more accessible. It has a performance rate of over 90 percent in patients, which is why more individuals choose it over gastric band procedure. Because you can do so in the safety of your own house as well, you don't have to think about the costs involved. Overall, it acts as a very easy way to tone down, decreasing the waste in nature. Again, no physical operation requiring intervention is used in hypnosis. It is a safe choice that lets you reach where you want to utilize creative and modern technologies. The hypnotherapy session includes visualizing the placing of a synthetic gastric band over your stomach that helps you to get the same feeling as you might initially have throughout surgery, but without the pain, unnecessary costs, and annoyance.

The result is that you feel like you are starving for longer stretches, need fewer calories, and feel whole, even though you have just consumed half of your regular-sized meal. This would also help you make better decisions and realize that a far better food experience than you presently have can be established. If you're curious if hypnotherapy for the gastric band would function for you, you should question whether you have the creativity to help your session. Everybody has an image now, of course, but is yours realistic enough? If you can shut your eyes and visualize staring at something that's not actually in front of you, then spend time reflecting on that, so you can effectively achieve so by gastric band hypnotherapy. Before you start something, it's natural to consider that it will struggle if it isn't adapted to you directly. Visual gastric band hypnosis will, however, provide emotional relief for you. This promotes your priorities, including weight reduction and improvement of fitness. When you invest time engaged in it, you can realize that you will accomplish whatever you put your purpose on. You will subconsciously erase your cravings, eliminate all detrimental and mental tension, as well as experiences that are part of your mental eating habit. Because impulsiveness forms a large amount of gaining weight, you can realize that it can be eliminated from your conscious mind and help any person willing to pursue it by hypnotherapy. As per a clinical report undertaken in the U.K., gastric band hypnotherapy has a 95% effective rate among patients. This analysis also found that certain patients would be willing to embrace and excel in hypnotherapy. Still, if they are not accessible to the experience, they will not find it useful. For a hypnotherapist's words to take action, individuals who are so cut off from fresh concepts, including hypnotherapy, sometimes made out to be a harmful activity by the uneducated, would not relax properly.

You'll know how it succeeds after only one hypnotherapy session since it is expected to start functioning after just one session. That is why all shouldn't get hypnotherapy. It is only recommended to someone prepared to shift their attitudes about food. It is called pointless if you do not trust it or bring you to where you want to go on your path towards weight reduction. Only after you have completed an appraisal will the expense of gastric band hypnotherapy services with a licensed hypnotherapist be determined. Energy stimulation strategies are often learned during these appointments and can also support any patient encounter with fear, frustration, tension, and all other harmful emotions.

CHAPTER 27:

Understanding the power of belief

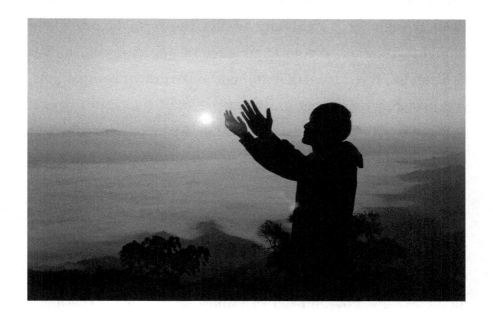

Belief and Believing

Beliefs are the thoughts valid to you. They may need not to be scientifically proven to realize them to be real for you. If you are aware of it or not, your movements, both conscious and subconscious, are functions of your beliefs. Even though your ideals are within the form of mind and thoughts, they shape your experience by affecting your moves in lifestyles. If you trust that animals make proper companions, you probably have a cat or dog or parrot or a ferret or two. If you agree with that coffee to continue with your conscious at night, you probably do no longer drink espresso before going to bed.

The electricity of believing helps you to affect your body in ways that might seem astounding. Placebo responses, where people reply to an inert substance as though it were the proper medicine, are not unusual examples of how we experience beliefs inside the body. If a person, in reality, believes that he will get well while taking a particular medicine, it will show up whether the tablet contains a remedy or is, without a doubt, inert. Identically, if someone without a doubt believes that he can achieve excessive grades in college, it'll appear. If someone believes that he can gain his best weight, it will manifest.

Remember your make-accept as real with games as a child. Your capacity to faux is just as sturdy now as while you had been very young. It can be a touch rusty, and you may want a bit of practice. However, while you allow yourself to be fake and believe in what you're pretending, you will find a powerful tool. You will discover that this is a wonderfully effective way to deliver your intentions, the ones with messages of what you need, to all the cells and tissues and organs of your body, which reply by bringing that purpose into reality for you.

We can't say this enough: thoughts are things. The thoughts, the pictures, and thoughts you put in your mind emerge as the messages your self-hypnosis conveys to your mind-body turn your ideal body into a truth. Pretending is choosing what to consider and turning into absorbed into one's ideas. Just as a magnifying glass can consciousness rays of sunlight, you could awareness your mental power to make your thoughts, ideas ideal for your shape.

Belief and Thinking

Whether you are mindful of it or perhaps not, your conscious and unconscious activities are based on the values of yours. Although your opinions are available in the shape of thoughts and ideas, they develop the experience of yours by changing the life activities of yours. In case you think that pets create beautiful companions, you more than likely have a dog or maybe parrot or cat or even a ferret or perhaps 2. In case you think that coffee will keep you awake during the night, you most likely do not drink coffee before you go to sleep.

The ability of thinking enables you to affect your entire body in a way that may appear astonishing. Placebo answers, where folks respond to an inert chemical as if they were the right medicine, are typical examples of how beliefs have been experienced within the body. If an individual believes he will become well when carrying a specific treatment, it will take place if the pill includes drugs or is only perceptible. In precisely the same manner, if an individual believes he can attain high school levels, it will occur.

If an individual believes he can reach his ideal weight, then it is going to occur. Recall your chosen matches as a kid. Your capacity to feign is equally as powerful now as if you're young. It Might Be a little rusty, and you may require a bit of exercise, but when you allow yourself to feign and think about what you're pretending, you will see a powerful instrument.

You will find that this can be a superbly productive method to produce your aims, these messages of everything you would like, to everyone the cells and organs and tissues of the human body, which react by bringing that aim in reality for you. We cannot state this enough: ideas are things. The ideas, the images, and thoughts you set in your head become the messages that your self-hypnosis communicates into a mind-body, finally turning your ideal body into a truth. Pretending is picking what to think and getting absorbed in these thoughts.

As a magnifying glass may concentrate beams of the sun, you can focus your emotional energy to create your ideas, thoughts, and beliefs actual for your physique.

Expectation

You might not always get what you would like, but you do get what you expect. Expectations include the power of faith, and eventually, become the outcomes of what's considered. Here's a good illustration of how to "expect." Once you sat down to read this novel, you didn't analyze the seat or couch to check its ability to maintain your weight. You simply sat down without even considering it.

You did not have to Consider It because a piece of your convinced, and contains so much religion in the seat, which you "anticipated" it to maintain you. That's the best way to anticipate the ideal body weight you would like. Bearing this in mind, be cautious of everything you say to yourself and others, seeing your body weight expectations. "I gain weight through the holidays" "Last evening I ate two pieces of cake, and this morning I had been just two pounds heavier."

Mind-Body in Focus

Every one of the vital ingredients may create powerful results when concentrated inside the mind-body. But when these ingredients have been calibrated correctly inside the self-hypnosis procedure, their efficacy has still magnified a hundredfold. Self-hypnosis is a procedure for making your reality. You may think that sounds magic or too fantastic to be correct, but that's relative to what you've got to this stage in your life. These thoughts may be relatively fresh for you. Here's a good instance of this "comparative" character of fresh thoughts.

Imagine that you're supplied a personal jet that's beautifully equipped with luxury appointments and also a well-trained crew. It's a fantastic gift, and you also get to reveal this technology marvel to some people who have not ever seen anything like this. Let's suppose your pilot strikes you back in time to before December 17, 1903, when the Wright brothers declared their first flight in Kitty Hawk. You're happy to reveal this miracle of technology to the Wright brothers, who come to greet you personally. What could happen? Maybe they'd be scared and would not think it is possible to fly into a metallic bird. You can give them a ride, and they may opt to run out of you. Folks can reject or resist new ideas, even if they're lovely.

Your subconscious (mind-body) utilizes the combo of everything you need (inspiration), everything you think, and what you anticipate as a blueprint for actions. The outcomes are attained by your mind-body (unconscious), rather than by studying or thinking. If somebody reaches a cold surface she thinks is quite sexy, she can generate a blister or burn reaction. Conversely, an individual touching a scorching surface, believing it is cold, might not create a burn reaction. Individuals who walk across hot flashes while imagining they are cool might undergo thermal harm (some slight scorching around the bottoms of the feet); however, their immune system doesn't react with a burn (blistering, pain, etc.) since their heads inform their bodies the way to respond. Again, it's the orientation of three of those vital ingredients which makes it easy:

- Desiring to take action

- Thinking it possible

- Hoping to become successful

The truth goes through three phases. First, it's ridiculed. Second, it's violently opposed. Third, it's considered to be self-evident.

That is the trick to achievement. Your entire body carries your own beliefs. Your beliefs guide your activities, which then form your expertise. Some explain this procedure as creating your achievement or producing your expertise in life.

In our civilization, we view this clarified within the inspirational and positive emotional attitude literature. It may be understood in several regions of metaphysics. It is also possible to look back at the ancients and watch what is explained in the historical period's details.

An individual much wiser than we're mentioned, "It'll be done unto you based on your view." In the current era of integrative psychology and medicine, we predict it self-hypnosis or mind-body medication. There continue to be many scientific studies that demonstrate surprising consequences for pain management, wound healing, physical change, and a lot more health benefits than we thought possible.

Choosing Your Beliefs

You can pick your beliefs. You might decide to think what you find, in the feeling of "See it to believe it" or even "Seeing is believing" That is pretty simple to accomplish. You encounter something together with your perceptions, and that's a comfortable manner of picking whether it's believable or not. However, you might also opt to think about it and then watch it, which might require some exercise. Many men and women find it simpler to allow the world to tell them what's accurate or what to think. The T.V, newspapers, media, novels, teachers, and specialists bombard us with everything to consider. You grew up learning about the planet and yourself from several outside resources. It also led to a recognizable routine of discovering and observing information concerning the earth from yourself, and you decided which advice to create part of your belief system. It comprised belief about your physique. As an instance, as soon as your belly produces a sound noise, you feel that means you're hungry. Or you are feeling nauseous and think you're sick. Both are examples of noticed events: you discovered a link once and decided to consider it. From the Rapid Weight Loss Diet," we're suggesting that you just turn that clinic around for this thought: "Think it, and you'll see it" It follows that you choose what to think, then your entire body works on it as authentic and which makes it real on your adventure. Among the important messages we expect that you will receive from that book is your mind-body hears that you hear, what you say, all you presume, imagine, or picture in your head, and it can't tell the difference between what's actual and everything you envision. It behaves upon what you would like, thinks, and hope. Remember, these statements would enable you to experience the ideal weight you want: "I only look at food and gain weight" or even "I will eat my weight remains the same"? Indeed, the latter. However, that statement do you believe to be authentic for you? Again, it is going to be done unto you based on your view. We'll help you with the thoughts, speech, and graphics that invent practical hypnotic ideas, but you need complete control of what you opt to trust. As you browse the tips in this novel and discover the hypnotic suggestions provided through the trancework about the sound, you may have many options. We wholeheartedly invite you to opt to think about it. You will notice it on your own. Your subconscious (mind-body) can't tell the difference and act on which you pick either manner. Why don't you decide what you want?

The Power of Emotions

Few ideas and beliefs manifest themselves in your expertise. Just the ones which possess the ability of your emotions (feelings), together with your perception and your anticipation that something will occur, will manifest themselves.

Your emotions or emotions are a Kind of energy which affects this procedure for creation. In other words, whenever you've got a strong feeling of a belief, then it includes energy. This energy generates your expertise and further strengthens your expectations and beliefs. We're speaking about your ideas' collective energy, beliefs, preferences, and what exactly you would like.

The psychological energy supports what you would like and just how much you allow yourself to desire; it generates inspiration. It's possible to observe it is crucial to let yourself want something with a good feeling. If you blend feeling with desire, you enable the procedure you're putting into motion inside you. Ensure your feelings stay optimistic. You can determine when they're negative or positive regarding how they make you feel. It is simple.

Emotions that cause you to feel good are favorable, and feelings that cause you to feel awful are unfavorable. Maintain each of these energies confident by feeling great about your needing (want), faith, and expectations. If you've got negative thoughts and emotions, then they'll harm your motivation. If you've got positive ideas and feelings, then they will fortify your motivation. Ideas, beliefs, and expectations will be equal-opportunity energies. You're able to bring them and create negative or positive results and results. If you're negative, then expect adverse outcomes. If you're positive, anticipate positive effects. In this way, any notion, opinion, or expectation produces a positive or negative result. It is a no-brainer--if you need success, seek good energy from positive ideas and feelings. Charles talked a litany of unwanted words. "My job is overpowering.

I don't have any opportunity to do anything but grow from bed in the morning, drive into the workplace, and attempt to keep everyone happy. I get a headache just thinking about my life. I cannot possibly consider losing weight; it's not in the film." Guess what? Charles gets upset all of the time, and that he continues to lose excess weight, and he'll do so until he quit having negative words to describe his life.

Choosing Your Feelings

Your mind-body also calms your perception according to your inherent sense. Here's a good illustration. Let's suppose you wish to think about something which can allow you to realize your objective. You write an affirmation and start saying it to yourself. Affirmations are an excellent means to produce positive suggestions and customs. Speaking affirmations enables your ears to listen to your voice. It also is a method of picking your beliefs and strengthening them. For Instance, you might say that the affirmation, "I'm thinner and lighter now." However, what would you believe? If you "feel" that you weigh too much or believe the affirmation is false and inform yourself of the affirmation anyhow, there's a battle. Everything you are feeling is just another way your subconscious mind your perception or hold as correct. Your feelings must be in working with your affirmations along with your desires, beliefs, and preferences. Remember, emotions (feelings) are all energy. You could be asking, "But what if I do not think what I am telling myself?" Can it anyway. It's far better than focusing on the power of your own emotions, needs, and faith in a negative way.

The Law of Dominant Effect

There's essential legislation about hypnosis, Known as the Law of Dominant Effect. It informs us that anything that dominates our idea, whatever modulates our perception, is what our bodies will act upon. So, if 51% of your brain considers "A," and just 49% of your brain feels "B," you will have "A," precisely what most, or even the dominance, your ideas are. It usually means you don't need to have utterly fantastic beliefs; you merely need to have the benefit of your opinion concentrated on what you would like. Indeed this is a situation where "better is better."

Time Is on Your Side

You don't need to be worried about just how long some routines or programs happen to be operating on your subconscious or mind-body. They could change the moment you find what Has to Be adjusted or realigned, in Addition to when you make the intentional option to alter them. We'd want you to be aware of how your mind-body comprehends time.

You're conscious of the mechanical and linear dimension of time in days, minutes, hours, and seconds--that which we call "clock time." That's the way your conscious mind knows the dimension of time. Your unconscious, you're mind-body, just knows "today time," at which one moment can look like ten, or even ten minutes may look like you, or what's occurring in the "now." On your sleeping, you can undergo a fantasy happening in the area you lived as a young child, but with individuals who went to a high school, folks you may notice in tomorrow's scheduled assembly, and also the individual who took your purchase for lunch daily. All this may happen at the Exact Same time in your fantasy, as your subconscious love all Moment as "now."

Throughout your trance work, you may discover Dr. G. mention your subconscious may use the hypnotic suggestions together with pictures and thoughts of their future as if they've already happened.

Considering that most of the time is "now time" for your subconscious, you can correct, substitute, or make the suggestions and programs which you would like to "conduct" in you "now."

CHAPTER 28:

Deep sleep meditation

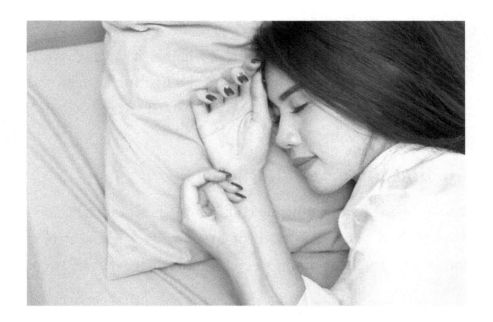

One of the best ways to relax and find the peace needed for better sleep is through a visualization technique. For this, you will want to ensure that you are in a completely relaxing and comfortable place. This reading will help you be more centered on the moment, alleviate anxiety, and wind down before bed.

Listen to it as you are falling asleep, whether it's at night or if you are simply taking a nap. Ensure the lighting is right and remove all other distractions that will keep you from becoming completely relaxed.

Meditation for a Full Night's Sleep

You are lying in a completely comfortable position right now. Your body is well-rested, and you are prepared to drift deeply into sleep. The deeper you sleep, the healthier you feel when you wake up.

Your eyes are closed, and the only thing that you are responsible for now is falling asleep. There isn't anything you should be worried about other than becoming well-rested. You are going to be able to do this through this guided meditation into another world.

It will be the transition between your waking life and a place where you will fall into a deep and heavy sleep. You are becoming more and more relaxed, ready to fall into a trance-like state where you can drift into a night of healthy sleep.

Start by counting down slowly. Use your breathing in fives to help you become more and more asleep.

Breathe in for ten, nine, eight, seven, six, and out for five, four, three, two, and one. Repeat this once more. Breathe in for ten, nine, eight, seven, six, and out for five, four, three, two, and one.

You are now more and more relaxed and prepared for a night of deep and heavy sleep. You are drifting away, faster and faster, deeper and deeper, closer and closer to a heavy sleep. You see nothing as you let your mind wander.

You are not fantasizing about anything. You are not worried about what has happened today or even farther back in your past. You are not afraid of what might be there going forward. You are not fearful of anything in the future that is causing you panic.

You are highly aware within this moment that everything will be OK. Nothing matters but your breathing and your relaxation. Everything in front of you is peaceful. You are filled with serenity, and you exude calmness. You only think about what is happening in the present moment where you are becoming more and more at peace.

Your mind is blank. You see nothing but black. You are fading faster and faster, deeper and deeper, further and further. You are getting close to being completely relaxed, but you are OK with sitting here peacefully right now.

You aren't rushing to sleep because you need to wind down before bed. You don't want to go to bed with anxious thoughts and have nightmares about the things you fear. The only thing you concern yourself with at this moment is getting friendly and relaxed before it's time to start to sleep.

You see nothing in front of you other than a small white light. That light becomes a bit bigger and bigger. As it grows, you start to see that you are inside a vehicle. You are laying on your bed. Everything around you is still there. Only when you look up, you see that there is a large open window, with several computers and wheels out in front of you.

You realize that you are in a spaceship floating peacefully through the sky. It is on auto-pilot, and there is nothing that you have to worry about as you are floating up in this spaceship. You look out above you and see that the night sky is more gorgeous than you ever could have imagined.

All that surrounds you is nothing but beauty. Bright stars are twinkling against a black backdrop. You can make out some of the planets. They are all different than you would ever have imagined. Some are bright purple, and others are blue. There are detailed swirls and stripes that you didn't know were there.

You relax and feel yourself floating up in this space. When you are here, everything seems so small. You still have problems back home on Earth, but they are so distant that they are almost real. Some issues make you feel as though the world is ending, but now that the entire universe is still doing fine, no matter what might be happening in your life. You are not concerned with any issues right now.

You are soaking up all that is around you. You are so far separated from Earth, and it's crazy to think about just how much space is out there for you to explore. You are relaxed, looking around. There are shooting stars all in the distance. There are floating rocks passing by your ship. You are floating around, feeling dreamier and dreamier.

You are passing over Earth again, getting close to going back home. You are going to be sent right back into your room, falling more heavily with each breath you take back into sleep. You are getting closer and closer to drifting away.

You pass over the earth and look down to see all of the beauty that exists. The green and blue swirl together, white clouds above that make such an interesting pattern. Everything below looks like a painting. It does not look real.

You get closer and closer, floating so delicately in your small space ship. The ride is not bumpy. It is not bothering you.

You are floating over the city now. You see random lights flicker on. It doesn't look like a map anymore, like when you are so high above.

You are looking down and seeing that gentle lights still flash here and there, but for the most part, the city is winding down. Everyone is drifting faster and faster to sleep. You are getting closer and closer to your home.

You see that everything is peaceful below you. The sun will rise again, and tomorrow will start. For now, the only thing you can do is prepare and rest for what might come.

You are more and more relaxed now, drifting further and further into sleep.

You are still focused on your breathing; it is becoming slower and slower. You are close to drifting away to sleep now.

When we reach one, you will drift off deep into sleep.

Sleep Well with Self-Hypnosis

This is going to be a thirty-minute guided hypnosis session to help you drift off into a deep and relaxing sleep. The most important thing to do while listening to this session is to keep an open mind. You must go with the flow, listen to my voice, and remember to breathe. Remember, it is not always possible to enter a light hypnotic state on the first try, but we will try as I guide you gently and smoothly into this state to fall asleep. Please bear in mind that you are not going to enter any sort of deep catatonic state. Nothing is going to be physically altered within the realm of your mind. The process of hypnosis and this guided meditation is exceptionally safe, and you are in control of it.

Now, I want you to get comfortable. Because you are trying to achieve deep sleep, you should be lying down, your head resting on your most comfortable pillow, and warmed by your softest blanket. Lie back and let your shoulders go slack, relaxing against the cushion of your bed. Gently close your eyes and release all the tension from your muscles. Release the tension in your arms, then your legs. Let go of the stress in your chest and your back. All of your body muscles begin to feel looser and looser, and your body is feeling light.

Recognize that this is a time for only you. You have set aside all of your day's activities and are ready to embrace a beautiful and peaceful sleep fully. Breathe in this moment of relaxation, where nothing else matters. There is only you in the warmth of your bed.

As you lay, I will ask you something very simple. In your mind's eye, imagination a kind of ruler or some sort of measuring device. Imagine something which can measure the depth of your relaxation. Imagine this ruler in front of your mind. Perhaps it is your favorite color, smooth with small painted tick marks and numbers.

Take a moment to notice where you are at your current level of relaxation, out of a scale of 100 down to 0 being your most relaxed state. Understand that there is no right or wrong measurement, to begin with. Explore your state, be honest with yourself as you measure your relaxation. What tensions do you still have left in your body? What anxieties, sadness, or pain still lingers? Very soon, you will increase your relaxation and melt away this negativity and drift off into a peaceful sleep.

Perhaps you are currently at a 60 on your scale of relaxation. Even though you may be lower down than that, imagine yourself moving the marker in front of you. With each deep breath, you slide the marker further down along this ruler closer and closer towards zero, towards immense relaxation. As you breathe and the marker slides down, you feel your muscles release in your arms, then your legs, your back relaxes, and your chest opens like a flower, welcoming in big and tranquil breaths.

You may be aware that your sense of relaxation has expanded inside of you. Perhaps down to 40 or 30. You see the marker slowly glide downwards along the scale. You feel that a wave of warmth has washed over you, and you are beginning to feel your whole body becoming engulfed in the warmth of peace. As you feel your body releasing its tension even more now, you feel calmer. You have now reached a ten on your scale, and gently, you take a deep breath through your nose. Let it fill your stomach until it is like to burst. Then release it.

You reach nine...You enter a peaceful, calm environment.

You reach eight...You can feel the warmth of the sun on your face. It is a reminder that you are loved.

You reach seven...Each sound that you hear, you do not deny. Instead, it lulls you further and deeper into a deep state of relaxation.

You reach six...You inhale through your nose and fill your belly. You inhale all of the good things the world has to offer.

You reach five...Gently, through your nose, you release your breath. You expel any negative feelings that remain.

You reach four...You feel your body becoming lighter. Your arms and legs feel weightless and free.

You reach three...You feel your chest brimming with warmth and light.

You reach two... You accept the peace that has enveloped you. This peace welcomes you into a deepening serenity as your mind quiets.

You reach one... You feel yourself drawn towards the warmth of peaceful sleep, so close you can almost graze it with your fingertips.

You reach zero... You feel a comfort deep within you that starts in your chest and radiates outwards like a blooming flower. This comfort fills you with security, and you remember that you are safe. You have released your worries and concerns, and in its place, there is warmth, light, and comfort.

Gently you are lulled by this wave of serenity. You feel yourself beginning to drift beyond zero, into a realm of warm colors. Billows of reds and pinks, yellows, and oranges undulate around you in soft embraces until you float down onto a plush, cool surface.

With only your fingertips, you detect that you have landed on a grassy field. Around you, you can smell the sweet fragrance of wildflowers that have populated this clearing. Your body and mind have quieted to listen to the soft rustle of the breeze through grass and flower petals, and you remember the beauty of the earth. You breathe in through your nose, a deep breath that fills your stomach. Through your nose, you slowly release it.

You recognize the warm colors from before, now painted in the sky. The reds fade into pinks seamlessly as though crafted by a painter's brush. The hues swirl into the setting sun and exude a warmth that you feel throughout your body. You exist in this space with only beauty. You live without concern for time or worry. There is only you in this space, and all of the tranquility it shares with you.

The pinks give way to magentas, then onto violets and dark blues. The sunsets and reveals an endless sky, sprinkled with thousands of twinkling stars. You see dustings of silver and purple in the sky. The bright sliver of the moon casts its beam upon you, cascading you in comfort.

Your muscles seem to melt, going slack, and welcoming sleep. The stars above you dance, twirling through the vast stretch of sky, but you are still. You allow this positive energy to enter your mind. It swells within you until you feel peace exuding from every pore. You have reached a depth of serenity that exists on the brink of sleep. Allow yourself to accept rest.

Underneath the moon, you accept rest. Soon, you begin to notice a new pleasing sensation that arrives at your arms and spreads to your legs and your back, your neck, and forehead. You recognize this sensation as sublime floating energy entering your body. You feel a delicate tingle throughout your body, ushering in lightness and calmness. This sensation is like soft white linen, cleansing you from the inside out. It is a warm touch of healing energy, love, and passion.

These soft vibrations rid you of tension. Anxieties are expelled. Sadness and fear no longer exist here. All of the excess stress is now dissolving entirely, turning into dust carried off by the wind. It is melting away under the power of this healing energy. In its place, there is safety and the knowledge that you are loved by whom you love. It is merely you, the stars, and the moon.

The lightness you feel swells as if tiny balloons are attached to different parts of your body. You feel your body beginning to rise and drift upwards in the direction of the stars. Peacefulness and serenity are lifting you higher into the air into the welcoming embrace of the expansive night sky. For a brief moment, you understand that you exist in the space between the earth and the sky, a realm that belongs to you and is safe from anxiety. You claim this realm as yours in which to dream. This is your dreamscape, where you float towards rest and sleep. Your realm is one of peace that connects the heavens with the ground. It is yours alone to govern, to allow only positive energy and love. You roam over the tops of trees, drift across the width of lakes, and coast above others, sleeping in their warm beds.

Your entire body now is floating higher and higher in this realm as you feel such joy inside as you realize you are now gliding through all of space. You are drifting and roaming here, no longer bound by gravity. You are now soaring like a hot air balloon, ascending higher and moving towards the infinity of this welcoming expansion. As you float, you are letting go of everything that you no longer need. You toss away unwanted negativity. You hold on to the comfort that peace grants you.

As you become just like the pure brilliance of the stars, a beautiful shining light, you feel your spirit break free, and finally, you can float out through the entire universe. You reach out further and further into the purest wisdom and the most loving embraces of all of the celestial beings surrounding you. They are calling you to rest, to dream, to sleep, to heal. You feel yourself realigning from within.

You feel yourself moving with tranquility and mindfulness, further and further. As you wade through the stars, you feel yourself gently feeling heavier. You understand that you are drifting towards rest.

You drift through the cosmos, feeling gravity's kind tug towards the ground. Gently you float towards the earth as a leaf falls from a tree, eager to meet its rest based below. You feel completely relaxed and slipping away into a restful sleep. Before you escape into your dreams, you return to your bed, where you are warm and protected. Your body softly nestles under the blankets, and your head snuggles into the pillow. You notice your arms and legs still feel weightless, and there is a residual warm vibration throughout, a pulsing that beseeches sleep. You happily oblige.

I am going to count down from five. When I reach one, you will fully embrace the peace that has engulfed you and lose yourself in sleep. You will feel yourself slipping into a calm and serene rest.

Five... You think of the night sky and its expansiveness. It melts away every remaining tension until your body and mind are relaxed. It is summoning your sleep.

Four... You feel the warmth of peace move from the top of your head and down your neck. It moves through your shoulders, radiates through your chest and stomach, and finally glazes over your legs.

Three... You feel your body become heavy, and you softly sink in a little deeper to your consciousness. You are safe and protected.

Two... You feel yourself drift away, like a leaf on a still pond. You float away quietly into the night.

One... You are now asleep, resting, and at peace.

Breathe in, breathe out. Breathe in, breathe out. When you wake, you will be refreshed and ready to take on the day. You will be prepared to conquer the stresses of your life now that you have conquered sleep.

CHAPTER 29:

A Lifelong Journey

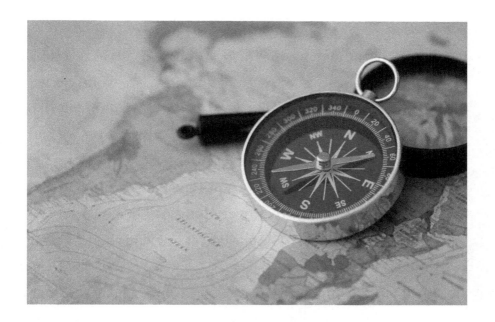

When we think about having to do something successfully, we often get caught up with the idea that we have to do things all at once. You have to pace yourself. If you're casually jogging instead of sprinting, then you're going to have a much lower chance of tripping and falling.

It will take just as long to change to a positive lifestyle as it took to get into a negative one. Unfortunately, we conditioned ourselves to think in a certain negative way. We often felt like we were not working toward our "success" or whatever we had defined it, as if we couldn't measure it in large tangible amounts. We have to start to look at the smaller things in life that can lead to success. Not everything has to be so big, so overdone. Instead, we can simply look at our jeans being a little loose on us as a massive milestone, rather than expecting to be able to fit into a much tinier size right away. Learn to take things in smaller amounts, and after a while, you will see the bigger picture.

We have to focus on methods that we can measure our success. Often, people will do this with numbers. They will hop on a scale, pull out a tape measure for their waste, or look at how quickly they might have been able to lose a certain amount of weight. None of this matter! You have to instead focus on the little milestones and how you feel overall. Sometimes, we measure success too much in ways that we think we can quantify. Everyone's journey will look different, including the victories we manage to make along the way.

You did your best; that's something that should be rewarded. If you can say that you honestly tried, then you should feel proud. You might not have gotten exactly what you wanted out of an individual situation, but you should still feel incredibly proud that you attempted something without giving up. As you move along your journey, your successes can get easier to measure, and you will also have larger goals. That is fine, though, because you will have the tools needed to achieve those more challenging goals.

CHAPTER 30:

Positive affirmations

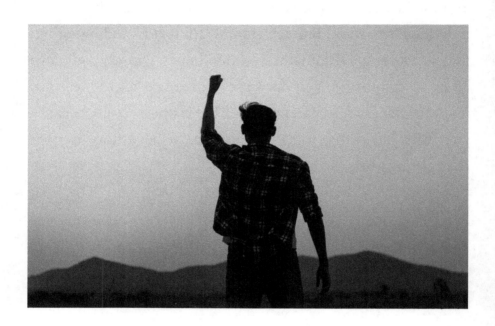

Thanks to my creator and everyone in my life.

I am grateful for all the bounty that I already enjoy

Every day I grow energetically and vibrantly

I only give my body the necessary nutritious food

My body is my temple

You can always maintain a healthy weight

I deserve to enjoy perfect health

Act to be healthy

I respect my body and am willing to exercise

My body is beautiful and healthy

I choose healthy and nutritious foods

I like to exercise, and I do it frequently

Losing weight is easy and even fun

I have confidence in myself

I am now sure of myself

I feel confident to succeed

From day today, I am more and more confident

I am sure to reach my goal

I want to be a noble example

I believe in my value

I have the strength to realize my dreams

I am adorable

I trust my inner wisdom

Everything I do satisfies me deeply

I trust the process of life

I can free the past and forgive

No thought of the past limits me

I get ready to change and grow

I am safe in the Universe, and life loves me and supports me

With joy, I observe how life supports me abundantly and provides me with more goods than I can imagine.

Freedom is my divine right

I accept myself and create peace in my mind and my heart

I am a loved person, and I am safe.

Divine Intelligence continually guides me in achieving my goals

Fear is a simple emotion that cannot stop me from succeeding

Every step forward I make increases my strength

My hesitations give way to victory

I want to do it, and I can do it

I am capable of great things

There is no one more important than me

That I can handle it

With confidence, I can accomplish everything

I allow myself to have a lot of fun

I deserve to be seen, heard, and shine

I deserve love and respect

I choose to believe in myself

I allow myself to feel good about myself and trust myself

I reduce measures quickly and easily

I can maintain my ideal weight without any problems

My body feels light and in perfect health

I'm motivated to lose weight and stay

Every day I reduce measures and lose weight

I fulfill my weight loss goals

I lose weight every day, and I recover my perfect figure

I eat like a thin person

I treat my body with love and give it healthy food

I choose to feel good inside and out

I feed myself only until I am satisfied. I don't saturate my food body

I know how to choose my food in a balanced way.

I feed slowly and enjoy every bite.

I am the only one who can choose how I eat and how I want to see myself.

It is easy for me to control the amount of what I eat.

I learn to have habits that lead me to my ideal weight.

Being at my ideal weight makes me feel healthy and young.

My body is very grateful and quickly reflects all the care I have for him.

My body reflects my perfect health.

I feel better every day

Being at my ideal weight motivates me to do other things that I like.

The human body is moldable, and I am the () artist of my body.

Every day I eat with awareness.

I consume the calories needed to have an ideal weight and a healthy body.

Every day I like the way I feel.

My slender body makes me feel agile, light (and) and healthy at the same time.

I know how to calculate the portions my body needs to feel adequately satisfied.

I can achieve everything that I propose.

No one can do this for me. Only I can make the best version of me, inside and out.

I am an inspiration for other people.

I like how the clothes look on my slender body.

I am strong, physically, and mentally.

No one can get me out of my motivation for being a healthy and slender person.

Being at my ideal weight fills me with energy.

My metabolism is faster every day thanks to the food I eat.

I love my new lifestyle.

I am getting better and better.

I accept all the blessings of the universe.

Reality is created from my thoughts.

I decide to choose thoughts that will have a positive impact on my life.

I am open to all new experiences of life.

I am free to think about what I want.

I will achieve great things.

I will be the best to accomplish this task.

I value myself because I am the right person.

I have full possession of my means.

I hide all the negative things that I cannot change.

I love myself a lot because I am the right person.

I can climb mountains.

I can reverse any reality.

I approve of everything I do.

All my decisions are taken in hindsight, and these are good for me.

I am unique.

I believe in myself inconsiderately.

I think positively.

Understanding is one of my most important qualities.

I have all the qualities in me to reach my ends.

I am determined to deal with all situations.

I am a man capable of exceeding my limits.

I am a unique person with great qualities.

I am the right person, and I deserve happiness.

All my decisions are good at different levels.

Serenity is an integral part of me.

Every day I weigh myself, the scales show significant weight loss.

Each day I successfully lose weight without fail.

My weight loss program is working like magic.

I have a happy and healthy attitude towards life.

I love my body; that is why I want the best for it.

My body is responding immensely to my weight loss efforts.

I can feel my body fats melting away.

I have developed a high rate of metabolism that helps me reach my ideal weight.

I have a complete focus on my weight loss journey.

When I set a goal, I make sure I achieve it.

Every day I wake up challenged and determined to reach my ideal weight goal.

No one and nothing can stop me from getting into the best shape of my life.

My determination to lose weight cannot be deterred.

My motivation to exercise is exceptional.

Every day I am motivated to follow a regular exercise regimen.

I am self-motivated and inspired to lose weight and follow a healthy lifestyle.

Being healthy is not only a lifestyle for me but a principle that I am determined to keep.

I choose to be a healthy and fit person.

I choose to eat healthily and maintain an active lifestyle.

I choose to feel fit and sexy.

My mind is hard-wired to want only healthy food, and my body automatically feels that need for daily physical activity.

My mind only accepts Positive thoughts and compliments about my body and resists any negativities that can divert me from my weight loss goal.

I am surrounded by people who help and motivate me during my weight loss journey.

I am worthy of good health.

I focus on positive progression.

I am a friend to my body.

I look after my body with unconditional compassion.

It feels good to exercise.

My metabolism is working to my advantage by helping me gain my optimal weight.

I am thankful for my body for all the things it does for me.

I know what to eat and how to live my life.

Every physical movement I make helps me maintain my ideal body weight.

The more I move, the better I feel.

My stomach is toned, my arms are toned I-am-in-shape.

I find it easy to stay in shape.

I'm grateful for my healthy, fit body.

I am in control of how the amount of food I eat.

Following a healthy eating plan is easy for me.

Eating healthy foods helps my body get all of the nutrients it needs to be in the best shape.

My metabolism is fast.

I acknowledge the beauty my body holds.

I believe in myself and acknowledge my greatness.

I bring the qualities of love into my heart.

I can accept myself for who I am.

Every day, I am getting closer to my ideal weight.

I am capable of achieving my goals.

I am happy about the feeling of wellness these changes are bringing me.

Every day, I increasingly love my body.

Trusting my body is becoming easier.

I stay focused on my ideal size.

This is my body; I treat it with respect and honor.

I am at peace with my body.

My body is being restored to its natural state of excellent health.

Love and affection flow into my life with ease.

I appreciate life.

All my wildest dreams and every good thing is flowing to me effortlessly and smoothly.

I'm entirely motivated to live a healthy life.

I have the power in me to make good things happen

I am becoming fitter and stronger every day through exercise.

I celebrate my power to make good and healthy choices around food.

I eat healthy meals.

Every day I am exercising and taking care of my body.

I am efficiently controlling my weight through a combination of healthy eating and exercising.

I maintain my ideal weight, and I enjoy life being fit.

I love the feeling exercising gives me.

I find time to exercise.

When I exercise, I feel powerful and alive.

I am burning calories every day.

I love exercising, and I love working out, I love eating natural foods.

It is easy for me to control my weight.

I love the taste of healthy food.

It's exciting to discover my unique food and exercise system for my ideal weight.

Everything I eat heals nourishes my body, and helps me reach my ideal weight.

I have a strong urge to eat only healthy foods and to let go of any processed foods.

I only eat nutritious foods, and I can easily resist temptations.

I am so grateful now that I have healthy eating habits.

Eating healthy comes naturally to me.

Healthy, nutritious food is what I eat every day.

My body benefits from the healthy food that I eat.

Healing is happening in both my mind and heart.

Healing happens with each step I take.

I quickly reach and maintain my ideal weight

I do what it takes to be healthy.

Every day I am getting slimmer and healthier.

I am a beautiful person inside out.

I can truly love myself for who I am.

I am grateful for the body shape I have been blessed with.

I accept myself for who I am.

I am grateful for the body I have.

I am getting closer to my ideal weight every day.

I am losing weight because I want to and because I have the power to do this.

Making changes is natural to me.

I am healthier and stronger with each day that passes.

Today, I focus on the good things that are unfolding in my life.

Every day is a new beginning.

I love my beautiful body.

I am content, peaceful, and full-filled.

I lovingly allow love, joy, and good health to flow through my mind and my body.

I am loved and am loving.

I am grateful for life and my body.

I am peaceful, joyful, and centered.

I believe in myself, and I will succeed.

I often visualize myself in my ideal weight

Exercising is fun, and it makes me feel outstanding.

I am happily exercising every day

I eat fruits and vegetables daily

Exercising is fun.

I am the person I think I am.

I agree with the people around me and trust my colleagues.

Self-esteem is my paramount quality.

My life is plenty of confidence.

I am a confident person who keeps getting better every day.

I trust my choices, and I move in that direction.

I erase in my life all the people who prevent me from achieving happiness.

I control my choices and my life.

I am responsible for my positive mental state.

I deserve a fulfilling life.

What I feel is healthy.

Trust in me is my first quality.

I attract good in my life.

I will offer everything I have given.

Love is present; it is enough that I believe in it.

I am aware that my friends love me.

I have a family and relatives who surround me.

I have a fulfilling social life.

I am in love.

I make the world better every day.

I like family time.

I take the time necessary to show my entourage how important they are to me.

I love them.

I can take time for myself and my loved ones.

Compassion is part of me.

I can give forgiveness.

I practice benevolence with conviction to help my entourage to evolve.

I can question myself and understand.

I choose to do what I like.

I believe in love.

I let my heart speak.

I can let people love me.

I like others, and others love me in return.

I accept that others can love me.

Fusional / passional love is coming into my life.

The people I love me back.

I can give love to others.

If I give others love, they make it exponentially.

I can attract the person I want.

My sentimental relationships are healthy and fulfilling.

I'm ready to fall in love.

I give a lot because I love this person

Love is in me.

Love is only an extension of my fulfillment.

Joy filled me and filled my life.

The people around me are filled with love, and I benefit from it.

I'm falling in love.

The waves around me tell me that love is present.

Hidden love is real love.

I love to love a person.

I take the front and reveal my love.

As a magician, I chose to give love all around me.

I like people, even my enemies.

I receive love as I pass it.

My life is happy and joyful.

I feel good with this person.

My relationship is passionate, and I feel fulfilled.

I give everything to my companion to make her as happy as possible.

Love is an integral part of my life.

Passion paces my choices.

I can let my heart make decisions.

My heart is full of happiness.

Harmony is present in me.

I love life, and life loves me.

I understand my feelings and accept them.

I deserve to find love

I am endearing and open to others.

I can open myself to others.

I can confess the things that I feel.

I only feel positive things about the people around me.

I only transmit positive to those around me.

I focus on the things that make me happy.

I believe in the power of attraction.

I concentrate my efforts on what I want.

Money is a reward.

I can get as much money as I want.

Money is a form of remuneration that takes different forms, and I am already rich.

CHAPTER 31:

Love your body

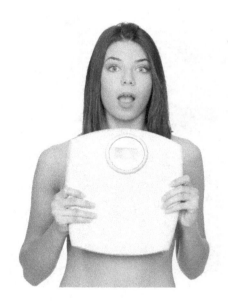

The majority of individuals don't think very much about self-improvement. We'd love to assist you in indulging in such a notion and finding out just how much you can enjoy yourself. It's a requirement to accept and create your ideal weight and everything else that's fantastic for you. Just being conscious of the idea of self-help can move you farther along on the way of enjoying yourself and accepting yourself as you are. Your character and character are aware of the way you're feeling on your own. If you harbor bitterness or remorse, or sense undeserving, these emotions operate contrary to enjoying yourself.

How can you see your flaws?

Can you blame yourself? Self-love and finding an error or depriving yourself repaint each other. It is tough to enjoy yourself if you frequently find errors ultimately.

Can you pay attention to the negative aspects of yourself?

Can you end up making self-deprecating statements, such as "I am not intelligent enough to..." or even "I am not great enough to..."?

Can you punish yourself or refuse yourself?

Can you establish boundaries with individuals who represent your very own moral and ethical criteria and your values and beliefs?

Look at the mirror. How do you feel about yourself? Can you smile or frown?

Which are you about the continuum of self?

Are you currently respectful and admiring?

Are you critical and judgmental, or would you love yourself for that you are?

Have you been cared for and caring for this individual who you see?

If you're ambivalent, then contemplate these concerns further. Be truthful with yourself. Have a conversation on your own. Take an honest look at yourself. Do not just examine your own body; examine your wisdom, your soul, your own emotions, along with your own heart. Know that: By enjoying yourself, you love yourself. If there's something that you can't accept on your own, be aware you could change that idea and alter it to make anything you want, such as your ideal weight.

How Does It Feel to Love Yourself?

Have a look at These features. Are these familiar to you? It is the way it should feel if you like yourself:

You genuinely feel happy and accepting your world, even though you might not agree with everything within it.

You're compassionate with your flaws or less-than-perfect behaviors, understanding that you're capable of improving and changing.

You mercifully love compliments and feel joyful inside.

You frankly see your flaws and softly accept them learn to alter them.

You accept all of the goodness that comes your way.

You honor the great qualities and the fantastic qualities of everybody around you.

You look at the mirror and smile (at least all the period).

Many confuse self-love with becoming arrogant and greedy. But some individuals are so caught up in themselves they make the tag of being egotistical and thinking just of these. However, we do not find that as a healthful self-indulgent character, which isn't well balanced in enjoying itself, love, and loving others.

It isn't selfish to get things your way; however, it's egotistical to insist that everybody else can see them your way. The Dalai Lama states, "If you do not enjoy yourself, then you can't love other people. You won't have the capacity to appreciate others. Suppose you don't have any empathy on your own. In that case, you aren't capable of developing empathy for others" Dr. Karl Menninger, a psychologist, states it this way: "Self-love isn't opposed to this love of different men and women. You can't truly enjoy yourself and get yourself a favor with no people a favor, and vice versa." We're referring to the healthiest type of self-indulgent, that simplifies the solution to accepting your best good.

Just take a better look at the way you see your flaws and blame yourself. Self-love and finding an error or depriving yourself aren't in any way compatible. If you deny enjoying yourself, you're in danger of paying too much focus on your flaws. That is self-loathing. You don't wish to focus on negative aspects of yourself, for by keeping these ideas in your mind, you're giving them the psychological energy which brings that result or leaves it actual.

Self-love is positive energy. Blame, criticism, and faultfinding are energy. Self-hypnosis can help you utilize your mind-body to make new and much more loving ideas and beliefs on your own. It helps your mind-body create and take fluctuations in the patterns of feeling and thinking that have been for you for quite a while, which aren't helpful for you. The trancework about the sound incorporates many positive suggestions to shift your ideas, emotions, and beliefs in alignment together with your ideal weight.

A Vital goal for all these positive hypnotic suggestions is the innermost feeling of enjoying yourself. If your self-loving feelings are constant with your ideal weight, it will likely occur with increased ease. But if you harbor bitterness or remorse, or sense undeserving, these emotions operate contrary to enjoying yourself enough to think and take your ideal weight. Lucille Ball stated it well: "Love yourself first and everything falls in line" The hypnotic suggestions about the sound are directions for change led to the maximum "internal" degree of mind-body or unconscious. However, the "outer" changes in life action should also happen.

Many weight reduction methods you have been using might appear to be a lot of work. We suggest that by adopting a mindset that's without the psychological pressure related to "needing to," "bad or good," or even "simple or difficult," with no judgment in any way, the fluctuations could be joyous.

Yes, even joyous. It produces the whole journey of earning adjustments and shifting easier. The term "a labor of love" implies you enjoy doing this so much it isn't labor or responsibility. The "labor" of organizing a family feast in a vacation season, volunteering at a hospital or school, or even buying a gift for someone very particular can appear effortless. Here is the mindset that will assist you in following some weight loss methods. We invite you to place yourself in the situation of being adored.

You're doing so to you. Loving yourself eliminates the job, which means it is possible to relish your advancement toward a lifestyle that encourages your ideal weight. Think about some action that you like to perform. Imagine yourself performing this action today. Notice that whenever you're doing something you love to perform, you're feeling energized and beautiful, and some other attempt is evidenced by enjoyment. At these times, you see it absolutely "loving what you're doing." Sometimes, we recommend that you also find that as "enjoying yourself doing this." Maybe by directing a more favorable attitude toward enjoying yourself, you'll end up enjoying what you're doing.

Giving Forth

Forgiveness is a significant step in enjoying yourself. At any time you forgive, you're "committing forth" or "letting go" of a thing you're holding inside you. Let's be clear about this: bias is simply for you, not anybody else. It's not a kind of accepting, condoning, or justifying somebody else's activities. It's a practice of letting go of an adverse impression that has remained within you too long. It's the letting go of any emotion or idea which can be an obstacle between you and enjoying yourself and getting what you desire.

A lot of us are considerably more crucial and much tougher on ourselves than others. When you continue to notions of what you should or should not have completed, you're not enjoying yourself. Instead, you're putting alert energy to negative beliefs about yourself. Ideas like "I should have obtained a stroll " or "I shouldn't have eaten this second slice of pie" can also be regarded as self-punishing. Sometimes, penalizing yourself, either by lack of overeating or eating, may even lead to a discount for your wellbeing. By shifting your focus to self-appreciation, you go from the negative to the positive, which is quite a bit more conducive to self-loving.

Writing in a diary about the wholesome choices you make every day may encourage self-improvement. By forgiving yourself and forgiving other people, you launch the psychological hold that previous events might have had on you, and you also make yourself accessible to appreciate yourself. When you launch the effects of earlier encounters by forgiving, you undergo reassurance and a calm comfort on your body, which helps you take your ideal weight.

You at the Head Table

Loving yourself involves placing yourself first. To drop fat and talk to the perfect weight of yours, you've to come. Therapist and writer Jean Fain wrote a post titled" The' Yes, I Will' Diet," originally printed in the 09/2005 issue of O: The Oprah Magazine. She recalls a forty-nine-year-old mum needed to drop pounds, telling her, "I do not care enough to care that I eat" She did not care about it in case she ate. She had not time for himself. Her life seemed to be in service that is constant to the demands of the husband of her, and the daughter of her, and her old mum, the company of her; they came. She ate junk food regardless of the weight reduction, taking blood pressure treatment, and the idea that a diet has been just a great deal, given her frame and plight of mind.

With her therapist's support, she found the time to hear relaxing CDs, find a massage, and see a book. Directly speaking, she discovered ways to put himself and tend to others with this high price itself. The article contained an email from twenty-five pounds lighter, saying, "I'm not at my goal yet, but I know that I shall succeed." Self-love and placing yourself go together. They're a winning combination. Any guilt you're feeling about putting yourself can be taken care of by fixing your reasons for feeling guilty and subsequently making decisions to eliminate them. Do anything is required to clean your path towards your ideal weight.

What Would You Like? What Do You Want?

Have you got a healthy self-image? There are lots of psychological tests that quantify self-image; however, our aim here isn't psychotherapy. So, let's just inquire, "Are you pleased with how you seem?" The question begs the following question: "What changes will please you?" There's no room for discretion, guilt, sorrow, or psychological energy to negative emotions. The questions and options are about what you'd like and exactly what you would like, followed by the ideas, beliefs, and activities that attract those outcomes around for you. Do you believe that your physical appearance influences how others treat you or feel about you?

Regrettably, the response for everybody is "yes." Body-size stereotypes are analyzed in many studies. Studies have shown that specialist therapists working with obese people have biases. If you're too heavy, you've felt that the others' prejudice throughout glances, ways of speech, and the differences in behavior toward you and the others of smaller size. Size-based discrimination could be hardest for children.

Along with the prejudice that kids have toward obese individuals is significantly rising. Research in 1961 reported that kids had discrimination against obese children. The study included revealing the kid's drawings and requesting them that they enjoyed the least. The four pictures portrayed kids, such as a kid in a wheelchair, yet a disfigured face, a person, known as "regular," and an obese kid. The drawing of this fat kid was chosen most frequently since the one that they enjoyed the least. This analysis was duplicated using 458 fifth-and sixth-grade kids in 2003.

In the new study, the difference between just how much they enjoyed the "ordinary" kid over the obese kid was greater than 40 percent higher than in 1961. Another study shows that adolescents who reported being teased about their weight have been dissatisfied with their bodies and considered attempted suicide. More Frequently than their peers who did not report being teased about weight.

These studies only validate that which any obese person perceives within our civilization. Overweight individuals don't require some reinforcement to dislike their self-image. The cultural and social biases and also body-size stereotypes produce debilitating feelings and might contribute to reducing self-esteem as well as weaker self-image. Evidently, at the social level, we will need to do a much better job of teaching ourselves about what's essential in valuing every individual and what's not. And we must approach problems of obesity using a more considerable sensitivity to individuals that weigh too much.

If you're experiencing difficulty with other people's glances and remarks about your body weight, use them to fuel your motivation to accomplish a wholesome body. Adopt the newest mindset, which each individual and each comment is presently a gift, not a curse. That's the way you should treat them as gifts. Each gift in the kind of an opinion about your weight is a reminder that you enjoy yourself, which you're moving toward your ideal weight, and that you're much more sensitive and compassionate than they are. Terry Cole-Whittaker composed a beautiful book titled Everything You Think of Me Is None of My Company. The publication title says everything and is a fantastic education about the best way best to

Conclusion

There are many reasons why someone should use hypnosis to lose weight. First, hypnosis is often successful when all other avenues of weight, health, and fitness have failed, and that's for a good reason!

The problem is not the method or even the plan you are using to achieve it. The problem is in your mind. If you want to lose real body fat, reduce weight, make your ideal shape, and maintain your new look, it is essential to change your attitude towards food and exercise and your behavior towards both.

The best hypnosis programs for weight loss may require you to understand and replicate those mental processes used by people who have lost weight already. It might be tough leaving your comfort zone. Hypnosis will help you reprogram your mind and install new thoughts that will become automatic habits once you identify the right behavior perfect for achieving your goal.

Eating less and adequately or exercise following a schedule won't be a dream anymore: hypnosis enhances and strengthens your will.

So, if you are worried about being overweight now, there is nothing wrong with undergoing hypnosis. After all, you have nothing to lose but weight.

Everything that comes from you that relates to you is just yours: your feelings, your voice, your actions, your ears, your thighs, your hopes, and your fears. That's why you are unique. Be happy that you are different from anyone, that you look the way you do and that it is just you. Start to feel that it's your own body, not something separate you need to live with.

Do you want your house to be just like anyone else's? Or do you love the little things that carry memories? Don't you love the atmosphere of your messy place after playing with your kids? And the plain curtain that you know you should replace, but which your mom sewed and looks so good? Or the piece of furniture that everyone says you should throw out, but you insist on it?

That's how you should feel about your body. You should understand that you don't need to compare it with anyone else's because it's impossible to compare unique things. Also, who determines what beautiful and ugly mean? You should not compare your body to the celebrities' perfect-looking bodies. First, because they are adjusted with Photoshop and other programs, and they are not real.

Ultimately, hypnosis, both in a professional or home setting, has the potential to help with weight loss. According to Vanderbilt University, hypnosis works best for individuals who need to lose low-to-moderate amounts of weight.

It doesn't mean that you shouldn't attempt it but talk with your doctor about working it into a routine that incorporates other weight loss behaviors. It requires a various number of hypnosis sessions by a hypnotherapist. It may take a long time before professional therapy alters your attitudes and actions, and it may take a while before changed behaviors become a habit.

Try not to get discouraged with little change. If nothing else, regular hypnosis sessions may help ease pressure and help you learn to relax, reducing your need to eat in emotional situations. Because hypnosis is probably not going to deal with the issue all by itself, consider keeping a food and exercise journal.

Also, record how long you practiced and what kind of activity you did. This log considers you accountable for poor decisions and allows you to distinguish patterns in your eating and exercise habits that may counteract healthy weight loss. When you identify these patterns, you'll have a venturing off point for your next hypnosis session, as far as critical thinking and behavior modifications may assist you with weight loss.

Regardless of how you approach hypnosis, its advantage may be what you have to finally lose that abundance of weight and carry on with a healthier life—good karma helps with using hypnosis to achieve your weight loss goals. Add up many small strides for weight loss success.

The more you practice the meditations we've given to you, the easier it will be to discover the success you've been waiting for. After a complicated diet, again and again, getting nowhere is an ideal opportunity to accept what isn't right about our mindset.

A perfect way to turn your mood around is to rework it through meditation. Tune in to these at whatever point you're home and find the opportunity. If you're exhausted, why not take a few minutes to relax and pull yourself together?

This meditation will be useful when you're feeling anxious. There may be a few evenings you may wake up and have trouble falling back asleep. Any one of these can help you relax while also encouraging you to fall into a weight loss mindset. Make sure you are placing yourself in a place where you can do these meditations safely.

Try not to drive with them, and regardless of whether you're taking a plane or other transportation where another person is in control, be cautious. When you do meditation, always do it at home in a safe place. Possibly, you will fall asleep without realizing it.

After you've attempted a few different reflections, you can use these methods on planes or anywhere else you may go if you know that you can stay awake and alert once you've come out of the meditation or hypnosis.

Recall that the meditations won't make you magically get more fit. They will help you get into the correct mindset necessary to finish the diet or exercise routine you are attempting. They will also assist you with relaxing and decreasing the pressure that can make this procedure harder.

Whatever strategy for eating healthy you may pick, these meditations and trances will help you stop gorging and think it is easier to eat healthily and practice naturally. Recollect that it takes over one attempt and that you should practice it regularly, not once a month. When you can incorporate these snapshots of relaxation into your routine, it will help them work better.

Good luck with your weight loss journey.

CPSIA information can be obtained
at www.ICGtesting.com
Printed in the USA
LVHW050052090221
678731LV00029B/1149